INTRODUCTION

In the quest for improved health and long-lasting weight management, many individuals embark on the transformative journey of gastric sleeve surgery. This life-changing procedure involves the surgical reduction of the stomach's size, empowering individuals with the tools to take control of their health and redefine their relationship with food. It's a decision that, while not without its challenges, holds immense promise and potential for a healthier, happier future.

Welcome to "The Gastric Sleeve Bariatric Cookbook." This cookbook is designed to be your trusted companion on your post-surgery path to a healthier, more vibrant you. It recognises the significance of gastric sleeve surgery in the grand scheme of weight and health management and its paramount role in guiding you towards success in your post-operative journey.

At its core, this cookbook aims to serve as a beacon of light, offering you a diverse array of delicious, nourishing recipes that align with the unique dietary needs and challenges that come with gastric sleeve surgery. It is our belief that a well-considered and satisfying diet can be a source of inspiration, empowerment, and strength on your path to recovery and long-term well-being.

Purpose And Promise:

The purpose of this cookbook is twofold: to provide you with a comprehensive, well-structured guide to post-surgery nutrition and to empower you with the means to create meals that are not only wholesome but also full of flavor. This book is your key to unlocking a world of culinary delights, each carefully crafted to meet your specific dietary requirements as you progress through the various phases of your post-surgery diet.

In these pages, you will find a wealth of high-protein, low-fat, low-sugar, and fibre-rich recipes to support your nutritional needs. Our aim is to make your culinary journey enjoyable and satisfying while also promoting your health and well-being every step of the way.

The Structure: What To Expect:

"The Gastric Sleeve Bariatric Cookbook" is organised to provide a seamless and progressive culinary experience. Each chapter is thoughtfully structured to guide you through the different phases of your post-surgery diet, from the early stages of clear liquids and full liquids to the eventual transition to solid foods. Within these pages, you will discover:

• Recipes tailored to the unique dietary requirements of each phase

• Nutritional information to help you make informed food choices.

• Guidance on portion control, hydration, and supplement management

• Meal planning strategies for creating balanced, satisfying menus

• Tips for navigating dining out and social situations with confidence

• A collection of personal success stories and advice from individuals who have walked the same path

As you embark on this journey of post-surgery recovery and long-term health, let "The Gastric Sleeve Bariatric Cookbook" be your trusted companion, supporting you in your pursuit of a healthier, more fulfilling life. Together, we can celebrate the joy of food, nourishment, and the transformative power of gastric sleeve surgery.

CHAPTER 1:

*Preparing for gastric
sleeve surgery*

A Brief Overview

Gastric sleeve surgery, also known as sleeve gastrectomy, is a popular and effective bariatric procedure designed to help individuals with obesity lose weight and improve their health. This surgery involves the reduction of the stomach's size, leading to a series of physiological changes that promote weight loss and metabolic improvements.

Here's a comprehensive overview of gastric sleeve surgery:

1. Procedure Description:

• During a gastric sleeve surgery, a portion of the stomach is surgically removed, leaving behind a smaller, sleeve-shaped stomach.

• The procedure is typically performed laparoscopically, involving small incisions and the use of a camera and specialised surgical instruments.

2. Weight Loss Mechanism:

• Reduced Stomach Size: The surgery reduces the stomach's

capacity, limiting the amount of food a person can eat at one time.

• Hormonal Changes: Gastric sleeve surgery also decreases the production of the hunger hormone ghrelin, which can lead to reduced appetite and food cravings.

3. Surgical Advantages:

• Compared to other bariatric procedures, gastric sleeve surgery is considered relatively straightforward, with a lower risk of complications.

• It does not involve the placement of foreign objects, such as gastric bands or adjustable gastric balloons.

4. Post-Operative Phases:

• Clear Liquid Diet: Patients begin with clear liquids immediately after surgery, gradually progressing to thicker liquids and pureed foods.

• Soft Food Diet: Patients then transition to soft, easily digestible foods.

• Solid Food Diet: Over time, patients reintroduce regular solid foods, albeit in smaller portions.

5. Benefits of Gastric Sleeve Surgery:

• Significant Weight Loss: Patients can experience substantial weight loss in the first 12–18 months post-surgery, often reaching a healthier body weight.

• Improvement in Obesity-Related Health Conditions: Many patients see improvements in obesity-related health issues, such as type 2 diabetes, sleep apnea, and high blood pressure.

• Enhanced Quality of Life: Weight loss often leads to improved mobility, self-esteem, and overall quality of life.

6. Considerations:

• Pre-Surgery Evaluation: Patients undergo thorough medical and psychological evaluations to determine their suitability for surgery.

• Lifestyle Changes: Successful outcomes require a long-term commitment to dietary and lifestyle changes, including portion control, regular exercise, and healthy eating.

• Potential Risks: While generally safe, gastric sleeve surgery carries risks such as infection, bleeding, and potential complications related to the surgery.

7. Long-Term Maintenance:

• Patients are encouraged to maintain regular follow-up appointments with healthcare professionals, including dietitians and support groups, to ensure ongoing success.

• Adequate hydration, vitamin, and mineral supplementation are often necessary to prevent nutritional deficiencies.

8. Non-Reversible:

• Gastric sleeve surgery is considered a permanent alteration to the stomach, as the removed portion cannot be reattached.

• This decision should be made with an understanding of its permanence.

What To Expect Before And After Gastric Sleeve Surgery

Before undergoing gastric sleeve surgery, it's crucial to understand what to expect both in the pre-surgery preparation phase and during the post-surgery recovery and adjustment period. Here's a breakdown of what you can anticipate before and after gastric sleeve surgery:

Before Surgery:

1. Pre-Surgery Evaluation:

o You will undergo a comprehensive medical evaluation to determine your eligibility for the surgery. This evaluation typically includes a physical examination, blood tests, and assessments of your overall health and readiness for the procedure.

2. Nutritional Counselling:

o You will receive guidance from a registered dietitian or nutritionist to help you make dietary changes before the surgery. This may include recommendations for a pre-surgery diet to reduce liver size and improve surgical safety.

3. Psychological Assessment:

o Some surgeons require a psychological evaluation to assess your mental and emotional readiness for the procedure. This is to ensure that you understand the surgery's implications and are prepared for the lifestyle changes it entails.

4. Pre-Surgery Diet:

o In the weeks leading up to the surgery, you may be placed on a specific pre-surgery diet that includes liquid or low-calorie meals to help you lose some weight before the procedure. This also reduces the size of your liver, making the surgery safer.

5. Educational Seminars:

o You may be required to attend educational seminars or support groups to learn about the surgery, the post-operative diet, and what to expect after the procedure.

6. Financial and insurance considerations:

o Ensure that you understand the financial aspects, including the cost of surgery, insurance coverage, and any pre-authorization requirements.

After Surgery:

1. Immediate Post-Surgery Period:

o You'll wake up in the recovery room, and medical staff will closely monitor your condition.

o Initially, you'll be on a clear liquid diet to allow your stomach to heal. You'll gradually progress to full liquids, pureed foods, and then soft foods before transitioning to regular solid foods.

2. Pain and discomfort:

o You may experience some pain and discomfort around the incision sites and in the abdomen for a few days. Pain medication will be provided to manage this.

3. Hospital Stay:

o Most patients stay in the hospital for 1-2 days after surgery to ensure a safe recovery. In some cases, you may be discharged sooner if you're recovering well.

4. Diet and Nutrition:

o You'll need to follow a carefully structured post-operative diet, which progresses from liquids to solids. Proper nutrition and portion control are essential for recovery and weight-loss success.

5. Hydration and Supplements:

o Adequate hydration is crucial. You'll need to take vitamin and mineral supplements to prevent nutritional deficiencies, as the reduced stomach size may limit nutrient absorption.

6. Physical Activity:

o You'll be encouraged to engage in light physical activity, such as walking, as soon as you're able to do so. Gradually, you can increase the intensity of your exercise.

7. Follow-Up Appointments:

o You'll have regular follow-up appointments with your surgical team to monitor your progress, address any concerns, and make adjustments to your diet or medications as needed.

8. Psychological and emotional support:

o Adjusting to the physical and emotional aspects of the surgery may be challenging. It's important to have access to psychological and emotional support, whether through support groups or individual counselling.

9. Long-Term Commitment:

o Remember that gastric sleeve surgery is not a quick fix. Long-term success depends on your dedication to lifestyle changes, healthy eating, and exercise.

Understanding the expectations and requirements before and after gastric sleeve surgery is essential for a successful and safe weight-loss journey. It's important to work closely with your healthcare team, including dietitians, surgeons, and support groups, to maximise the benefits of the surgery and ensure your long-term well-being.

Suggested pre-surgery dietary changes and meal planning.

Pre-surgery dietary changes and meal planning are essential to preparing your body for gastric sleeve surgery. These changes aim to reduce the size of your liver, make the surgery safer, and help you adapt to the post-surgery diet more easily. Here are some suggested pre-surgery dietary changes and meal planning guidelines:

1. Start Early:

• Begin making dietary changes several weeks before your scheduled surgery date to maximise the benefits.

2. High-Protein Diet:

• Focus on a high-protein, low-carbohydrate diet to help you lose weight and reduce liver size.

• Include lean protein sources like chicken, turkey, fish, lean cuts of beef, tofu, and low-fat dairy products.

3. Avoid sugary and processed foods.

• Eliminate or significantly reduce sugary beverages,

sweets, and highly processed foods.

• Minimise your intake of sugary snacks and high-carb, low-nutrient foods.

4. Portion Control:

• Practice portion control to get used to eating smaller meals. Use smaller plates to visually control portions.

• Avoid overeating and take time to savour your food.

5. Hydration:

• Stay well-hydrated by drinking plenty of water. Proper hydration is essential for overall health and will be important post-surgery as well.

6. Avoid alcohol and caffeine.

• Reduce or eliminate alcohol and caffeine consumption as part of your pre-surgery preparations.

7. Nutrient-Rich Foods:

• Consume nutrient-dense foods like fruits, vegetables, and whole grains to ensure your body receives essential vitamins and minerals.

8. Vitamin and mineral supplements:

• Talk to your healthcare provider about any vitamin and mineral supplements you should be taking before the surgery to address any nutritional deficiencies.

9. Pre-Surgery Diet Plan:

• Work with a registered dietitian or nutritionist to create a pre-surgery diet plan tailored to your specific needs and health status.

• A typical pre-surgery diet may include a combination of high-protein shakes, lean protein, and low-carb, low-sugar vegetables.

10. Gradual Changes:

• Avoid crash diets or extreme calorie restrictions, as these can be counterproductive and may be harmful.

• Instead, aim for gradual, sustainable changes in your eating habits.

11. Avoid Fried and Fatty Foods:

• Steer clear of fried and high-fat foods, as these can be hard on the liver and digestive system.

12. Emotional Preparation:

• Use this time to prepare mentally and emotionally for the changes that come with the surgery and the post-surgery lifestyle.

13. Record Your Progress:

• Keep a food journal to track your dietary changes and measure your progress. This can also help you identify areas for improvement.

14. Stay Compliant:

• Adherence to your pre-surgery diet and lifestyle changes is crucial. It will not only prepare you physically but also demonstrate your commitment to the surgery to your healthcare team.

CHAPTER 2:

*Gastric Sleeve Surgery
Nutritional Approach*

Nutrition is a critical aspect of the gastric sleeve surgery journey. After undergoing this procedure, it's essential to make informed dietary choices to promote healing, achieve weight loss goals, and maintain long-term health.

Here's an overview of the key nutritional considerations for individuals who have had gastric sleeve surgery:

1. High-Protein Diet:

• Protein is a primary focus post-surgery. It helps with tissue healing, muscle preservation, and satiety.

• Lean protein sources include chicken, turkey, fish, lean cuts of beef, tofu, low-fat dairy, and plant-based proteins like beans and lentils.

2. Portion Control:

• A smaller stomach means smaller portion sizes. Be mindful of portion control to prevent overeating and discomfort.

• Use small plates, bowls, and utensils to help manage portion sizes visually.

3. Balanced Meals:

• Aim for balanced meals that include protein, vegetables, and whole grains.

• Prioritize nutrient-dense foods to meet your nutritional needs.

4. Avoid sugary and high-fat foods.

• Minimize or eliminate sugary snacks, high-calorie beverages, and highly processed foods.

• Avoid fried and fatty foods, as they can be challenging to digest and may lead to discomfort.

5. Stay Hydrated:

• Maintain proper hydration by sipping water throughout the day. Dehydration can be a concern due to the reduced stomach capacity.

• Avoid drinking with meals, as it may fill you up too quickly and limit nutrient intake.

6. Fiber-Rich Foods:

• Gradually incorporate fiber-rich foods, such as fruits, vegetables, and whole grains, to support digestion.

• Be cautious with high-fiber foods in the early post-surgery phases, as they may be harder to tolerate.

7. Vitamin and mineral supplements:

• Gastric sleeve surgery may lead to nutritional deficiencies. You'll need to take vitamin and mineral supplements to prevent them.

• Common supplements include multivitamins, calcium, vitamin D, and vitamin B12, among others.

8. Gradual Progression:

• Follow the recommended post-surgery diet phases, progressing from clear liquids to regular solid foods under the guidance of your healthcare team.

9. Avoid carbonated beverages.

• Carbonated beverages can cause discomfort and gas. It's best to avoid them.

10. Emotional Eating Awareness:

• Pay attention to emotional eating and establish healthy coping mechanisms to avoid overeating.

11. Mindful Eating:

• Practice mindful eating by savoring each bite, chewing thoroughly, and eating slowly to prevent discomfort and promote digestion.

12. Regular Follow-Up:

• Maintain regular follow-up appointments with your healthcare team, including dietitians, to monitor your nutritional status and adjust your diet or supplements as needed.

13. Long-Term Commitment:

• Understand that gastric sleeve surgery is not a one-time solution; it requires a long-term commitment to a healthy lifestyle, including regular exercise and a balanced diet.

Foods To Eat And Avoid

After gastric sleeve surgery, it's essential to be mindful of the foods you eat to promote healing, prevent complications, and achieve your weight loss and health goals. Here's a general guideline on foods to eat and foods to avoid:

Foods to Eat:

1. High-Protein Foods:

o Lean meats (e.g., chicken, turkey, fish)

o Lean cuts of beef

o Pork loin

o Tofu

o Eggs

o Low-fat dairy products

o Plant-based proteins (e.g., beans, lentils, and quinoa)

2. Non-Starchy Vegetables:

o Leafy greens (e.g., spinach, kale)

o Broccoli

o Cauliflower

o Bell peppers

o Tomatoes

o Zucchini

o Cucumbers

3. Whole Grains:

o Oatmeal

o Brown rice

o Quinoa

o Whole-wheat pasta (in moderation)

o Whole-grain bread (in moderation)

4. Fruits (in moderation):

o Choose fruits with a lower sugar content, such as berries, apples, and citrus fruits.

o Consume fruit in small portions due to the sugar content.

5. Dairy (in moderation):

o Low-fat or non-fat dairy options, such as Greek yogurt or skim milk,

o Be cautious with dairy, as it can be high in calories and may cause discomfort.

6. Healthy Fats:

o Avocado (in moderation)

o Nuts (in moderation)

o Olive oil (used sparingly)

7. Nutrient-Dense Snacks:

o Greek yogurt

o Hummus with raw vegetables

o Nuts (in moderation)

o Nut butter (in moderation)

8. Hydration:

o Water is the best choice. Drink plenty of it to stay hydrated.

o Herbal teas (non-caffeinated) are also a good option.

o Sip fluids throughout the day, but avoid drinking with meals.

Foods to avoid:

1. Sugary foods and beverages:

o Soda

o Candy

o Sugary snacks

o High-sugar cereals

2. High-Fat and Fried Foods:

o Deep-fried foods

o High-fat meats

o Butter, margarine, and excessive oil

3. Carbonated Beverages:

o Carbonated drinks can cause gas and discomfort, so it's best to avoid them.

4. Tough and Fibrous Foods:

o Foods like tough cuts of meat, raw vegetables, and certain fruits with skins can be difficult to digest, especially in the early stages of recovery.

5. Large Portions:

o Due to the reduced stomach size, be cautious about portion sizes. Smaller, more frequent meals are recommended.

6. Alcohol:

o Alcohol can be rapidly absorbed and may have a stronger effect on those who have had gastric sleeve surgery. It's best to avoid it or consume it in moderation.

7. Caffeine:

o Limit caffeine intake, as it can irritate the stomach lining.

8. Processed and High-Sodium Foods:

o Foods high in salt, additives, and preservatives should be minimized.

Post-Surgery Diet Phases

The post-surgery diet for gastric sleeve patients typically consists of several progressive phases, each designed to allow the stomach to heal and gradually reintroduce solid foods. Here's a detailed overview of the different phases of the post-surgery diet:

1. Clear Liquid Phase:

• Immediately after surgery, patients start with clear liquids.

• These include:

o Water

o Clear broth (low-sodium)

o Sugar-free gelatin

o Sugar-free, non-carbonated beverages

o Clear fruit juices (diluted and low in sugar)

• The primary goal of this phase is to stay hydrated while avoiding any solid or opaque liquids that may irritate the stomach.

2. Full Liquid Phase:

• During this phase, you can start incorporating thicker, high-protein liquids for added nutrition.

• Approved full liquids include:

o Protein shakes or protein-fortified beverages

o Cream-based soups (strained)

o Low-fat, sugar-free yogurt

o Milk or milk alternatives (unsweetened)

• This phase ensures that you continue to meet your protein and nutritional requirements as your body heals.

3. Pureed Food Phase:

• In this phase, you transition to pureed or blended foods, which have a consistency similar to baby food.

• Suitable foods may include:

o Pureed lean meats (chicken, turkey, and lean beef)

o Mashed or pureed vegetables (e.g., carrots, sweet potatoes)

o Cottage cheese

o Unsweetened applesauce

• It's important to avoid any chunks or solid pieces during this phase.

4. Soft Food Phase:

• Now you can introduce soft, easily digestible foods with a bit more texture.

• Options include:

o Scrambled eggs or egg substitute

o Mashed potatoes (no added butter)

o Well-cooked, finely diced, or ground meats

o Cooked, soft vegetables (avoid skins and fibrous parts)

• Continue to avoid tough or fibrous foods that may be hard

to digest.

5. Transition to a Regular Diet:

• Over time, you'll gradually reintroduce regular solid foods into your diet.

• Focus on foods that are well tolerated and easy to digest, gradually expanding your food choices.

• Always chew your food thoroughly to prevent discomfort and support digestion.

Key points to remember:

• Portion control is crucial throughout all phases of the post-surgery diet to avoid overeating.

• High-protein foods should remain a priority to support healing and maintain muscle mass.

• Hydration is essential; aim to sip water throughout the day.

• Avoid carbonated beverages, as they can cause discomfort and gas.

• Focus on nutrient-dense foods, such as lean proteins, vegetables, and whole grains, as you transition to a regular diet.

• Continue to take any prescribed vitamin and mineral supplements to prevent nutritional deficiencies.

Dietary Recommendations

Dietary recommendations for individuals who have undergone gastric sleeve surgery focus on high-protein, low-fat, low-sugar, and nutrient-dense foods, with an emphasis on portion control. Here are some dietary recommendations, along with examples of recipes and their ingredients for different post-surgery phases:

1. Clear Liquid Phase (Days 1–7):

• Clear liquids are essential to maintain hydration and ease digestion during the initial recovery phase. This phase generally includes:

Recipe Example: Clear Chicken Broth

• Ingredients:

o Low-sodium chicken broth

o Water

Instructions:

• Heat the chicken broth and water in a pot.

• Sip slowly to avoid overfilling the stomach.

2. Full Liquid Phase (Days 8–14):

• In this phase, you can incorporate high-protein liquids and slightly thicker options.

Recipe Example: Protein Shake

• Ingredients:

o Protein powder (unflavored or low-sugar)

o Unsweetened almond milk or water

o A small amount of nut butter (optional)

o Ice cubes

Instructions:

• Blend all the ingredients until smooth.

• Adjust the thickness by adding more or less liquid.

3. Pureed Food Phase (Weeks 3–4):

• During this phase, you can introduce pureed or blended foods.

Recipe Example: Butternut Squash Puree

• Ingredients:

o Butternut squash, peeled and cubed

o Low-sodium vegetable or chicken broth

o A pinch of nutmeg

o Salt and pepper to taste

Instructions:

• Cook the butternut squash in broth until soft.

• Blend the cooked squash with nutmeg, salt, and pepper until smooth.

4. Soft Food Phase (Weeks 5–6):

• As you transition to soft foods, you can incorporate more texture into your meals.

Recipe Example: Scrambled Eggs with Spinach

• Ingredients:

o Scrambled eggs (2 eggs)

o Fresh spinach, chopped

o A small amount of low-fat cheese (optional)

o Salt and pepper to taste

Instructions:

• Scramble the eggs and fold in the spinach and cheese.

• Season with salt and pepper.

5. Transition to a Regular Diet (Week 7 and Beyond):

• As you progress, you can reintroduce regular solid foods while maintaining smaller portions and a focus on nutrient-dense options.

Recipe Example: Grilled Chicken Salad

• Ingredients:

o Grilled chicken breast, sliced

o Mixed greens

o Cherry tomatoes

o Cucumber

o Balsamic vinaigrette (in moderation)

Instructions:

• Toss the ingredients together and drizzle with a small amount of vinaigrette.

Important Tips:

• Chew thoroughly. Chew your food well to facilitate digestion.

• Portion control: Use smaller plates and utensils to help control portion sizes.

• Stay hydrated: Sip water throughout the day, but avoid drinking with meals.

• Monitor sugar and fat intake: Be mindful of the sugar and fat content of your food choices.

• Nutrient-dense choices: Prioritize lean proteins, vegetables, and whole grains to meet your nutritional needs.

Sample meal plans for each phase

Meal planning and timing during each phase of the postgastric sleeve surgery diet are crucial for a successful recovery and weight loss journey. Here are sample meal plans and timing guidelines for each phase:

1. Clear Liquid Phase (Days 1–7):

• During this phase, your primary focus is on staying hydrated and allowing your stomach to heal. You will consume clear liquids in small amounts throughout the day.

Sample Meal Plan:

• Morning: Clear chicken broth

• Mid-morning: sugar-free gelatin

• Lunch: Clear vegetable broth

• Afternoon: sugar-free popsicle or ice chips

• Dinner: Clear beef broth

• Evening: sugar-free, non-carbonated beverage

2. Full Liquid Phase (Days 8–14):

• In this phase, you can introduce thicker, high-protein liquids while continuing to prioritize hydration.

Sample Meal Plan:

• Breakfast: Protein shake (protein powder, almond milk, or water)

• Mid-morning: Greek yogurt (unsweetened)

• Lunch: cream-based soup (strained)

• Afternoon: Protein shake or protein-fortified beverage

• Dinner: low-fat milk or milk alternative (unsweetened)

• Evening: sugar-free, non-carbonated beverage

3. Pureed Food Phase (Weeks 3–4):

• This phase allows you to introduce pureed or blended foods with a consistency similar to baby food. Aim for high-protein options.

Sample Meal Plan:

• Breakfast: Scrambled eggs (2 eggs) with mashed avocado

• Mid-morning: Cottage cheese (low-fat)

• Lunch: pureed chicken or turkey with pureed sweet potatoes

• Afternoon: Pureed vegetables (e.g., carrots or peas)

• Dinner: low-sugar applesauce

• Evening: sugar-free, non-carbonated beverage

4. Soft Food Phase (Weeks 5–6):

• In this phase, you can start incorporating soft, easily digestible foods with more texture.

Sample Meal Plan:

• Breakfast: Greek yogurt with honey

• Mid-morning: Soft scrambled eggs with finely diced vegetables

• Lunch: Mashed potatoes (without added butter) with ground turkey

• Afternoon: cooked and finely diced vegetables (e.g., green beans)

• Dinner: Low-sugar fruit (e.g., canned peaches)

• Evening: sugar-free, non-carbonated beverage

5. Transition to a Regular Diet (Week 7 and Beyond):

• As you transition to a regular diet, you can reintroduce a wider variety of foods while maintaining smaller portion sizes and a focus on nutrient-dense options.

Sample Meal Plan:

• Breakfast: scrambled eggs with spinach and a side of whole-grain toast (in moderation)

• Mid-morning: Greek yogurt with fresh berries

• Lunch: Grilled chicken salad with mixed greens, cherry tomatoes, and cucumber

• Afternoon: Almonds (in moderation)

• Dinner: Baked salmon with steamed broccoli and quinoa

• Evening: sugar-free, non-carbonated beverage

Important Tips:

• Portion control: Continue to eat smaller, well-balanced meals throughout the day.

• Chew thoroughly. Take your time with each bite to support digestion.

• Hydration: Sip water between meals to ensure proper hydration.

• Monitor sugar and fat intake: Be mindful of the sugar and fat content of your food choices.

• Nutrient-dense choices: Prioritize lean proteins,

vegetables, and whole grains to meet your nutritional needs.

CHAPTER 3:

High-Protein Recipes

Clear Liquid Phase:

Protein-Rich Clear Broth

Ingredients:

• 2 cups of low-sodium chicken or vegetable broth

• 1 scoop (approximately 10-15 grams) unflavored protein powder

Step-by-Step Instructions:

1. In a saucepan, heat the low-sodium chicken or vegetable broth over medium heat. You can use store-bought or homemade broth, but ensure it is low in sodium to prevent excessive salt intake.

2. While the broth is heating, measure out one scoop of unflavored protein powder. It's essential to use a high-quality protein powder recommended by your healthcare team or dietitian.

3. Once the broth begins to simmer but not boil, carefully add the unflavored protein powder to the saucepan. Be sure to whisk continuously to prevent clumps and ensure the protein powder dissolves completely.

4. Continue to heat the broth and protein powder mixture

for another 2-3 minutes, stirring occasionally. Ensure that the broth does not come to a boil, as this may affect the consistency.

5. Remove the saucepan from the heat, and let it cool slightly before serving. The broth should be clear and protein-rich, providing essential nutrients without any solid pieces.

Portion Sizes:

• This recipe yields approximately two servings of protein-rich clear broth. Each serving consists of 1 cup of the prepared broth, making it easier to manage portion control during the clear liquid phase following gastric sleeve surgery.

Cooking Methods:

• The cooking method used in this recipe is stovetop heating. It's essential to avoid boiling the broth, as this can negatively impact the consistency and protein content. Simmer the broth to heat it gently.

Storage and Reheating:

• To store any leftover broth, let it cool to room temperature and transfer it to an airtight container. Refrigerate the broth for up to 3-4 days. When reheating, do so gently on the stovetop or in the microwave, ensuring it doesn't come to a boil.

Nutritional Information (per serving):

• Calories: Approximately 45-60 calories per serving, depending on the specific protein powder and broth used.

• Protein: Approximately 10-15 grams of protein per serving.

• Sodium: Less than 100 milligrams of sodium per serving with low-sodium broth.

• Fat: Minimal to no fat content.

• Carbohydrates: Minimal to no carbohydrates.

Health Benefits:

• This protein-rich clear broth is tailored to meet the nutritional needs of individuals in the early post-surgery phases. It provides essential protein to support healing and recovery, especially when solid foods are limited. The low-sodium content helps prevent excessive salt intake, which can be detrimental after gastric sleeve surgery. Additionally, this clear broth is easy to digest and gentle on the stomach, making it an ideal choice during the clear liquid phase. It offers a convenient way to meet protein requirements while adhering to dietary guidelines.

Protein-Infused Jello

Ingredients:

• 1 packet (0.3 oz or 8 g) of sugar-free gelatin (any flavor of your choice)

• 1 scoop (approximately 10-15 grams) unflavored protein powder

• 1 cup of water

Step-by-Step Instructions:

1. In a heatproof mixing bowl, combine the sugar-free gelatin powder and unflavored protein powder. Mix them together until well combined.

2. In a separate microwave-safe container, heat 1 cup of

water until it's hot but not boiling. You can heat the water in the microwave for about 1-2 minutes or use a kettle to heat the water separately.

3. Carefully pour the hot water into the bowl with the gelatin and protein powder mixture. Stir continuously until all the powder is fully dissolved and the mixture becomes smooth. This should take about 2-3 minutes.

4. Allow the mixture to cool for a few minutes to avoid denaturing the protein. During this time, you can skim off any foam or bubbles that may have formed on the surface.

5. Once the mixture has cooled slightly, pour it into your desired molds or a glass dish. You can use silicone molds or a shallow dish, depending on the shapes you prefer for your Jello. Place the molds or dish in the refrigerator.

6. Allow the Jello to set in the refrigerator for at least 3-4 hours, or until it is firm and has a gel-like consistency.

7. Once the Protein-Infused Jello has set, remove it from the molds or cut it into cubes if you used a dish.

8. Serve chilled and enjoy your protein-infused treat!

Portion Sizes:

• This recipe typically yields 2-4 servings, depending on the size of your molds or the dish you use. Each serving is equivalent to the portion size of one Jello mold or a portion cut from the dish.

Cooking Methods:

• This recipe primarily involves mixing, pouring, and refrigerating. No additional cooking methods are required.

Storage and Reheating:

• Leftover Protein-Infused Jello can be stored in an airtight container in the refrigerator for up to 3-4 days. There is no need for reheating. Simply serve it chilled.

Nutritional Information (per serving):

• Calories: Approximately 20-30 calories per serving, depending on the specific brand of sugar-free gelatin and protein powder used.

• Protein: Approximately 7-10 grams of protein per serving.

• Carbohydrates: Minimal to no carbohydrates, as it's sugar-free.

• Fat: Minimal to no fat content.

Health Benefits:

• This Protein-Infused Jello is designed to provide a protein boost while offering a tasty and low-calorie treat. It's a suitable option for individuals in the post-surgery phases who need to meet their protein intake goals without consuming a lot of calories or carbohydrates. The use of unflavored protein powder ensures that the Jello maintains its gelatinous texture while adding a protein element to the dessert. The sugar-free aspect aligns with dietary recommendations to limit added sugars, making it an excellent choice for bariatric patients. It's an enjoyable way to incorporate more protein into the diet, contributing to healing and muscle preservation during the recovery process.

Full Liquid Phase:

High-Protein Fruit Smoothie

Ingredients:

• 1 cup unsweetened almond milk

• 1 scoop (approximately 10-15 grams) unflavored protein powder

• 1/2 cup frozen mixed berries (e.g., strawberries, blueberries, raspberries)

• 1/2 cup unsweetened Greek yogurt

Step-by-Step Instructions:

1. Start by adding the unsweetened almond milk to your blender. It serves as the liquid base for your smoothie.

2. Next, add the unflavored protein powder to the almond milk in the blender. This will be your primary protein source, and it's essential for those in the post-bariatric surgery phases.

3. Toss in the frozen mixed berries. These provide natural sweetness and essential nutrients, such as antioxidants and fiber.

4. Add the unsweetened Greek yogurt to the mix. Greek yogurt is high in protein and adds a creamy texture to the smoothie.

5. Secure the blender's lid and blend all the ingredients on high speed until the mixture is smooth and creamy. This usually takes about 30-60 seconds, depending on your blender's power.

6. Once the smoothie is well-blended, pour it into a glass.

7. Enjoy your delicious and protein-packed fruit smoothie!

Portion Sizes:

• This recipe yields one serving of a high-protein fruit

smoothie.

Cooking Methods:

• The cooking method used in this recipe is blending. There is no need for additional cooking.

Storage and Reheating:

• Ideally, you should consume the smoothie immediately to enjoy its freshness. However, if you have leftovers, you can store them in the refrigerator for a short time, and give it a quick stir before consuming.

Nutritional Information (per serving):

• Calories: Approximately 200-250 calories per serving, depending on the specific brand of almond milk, protein powder, and yogurt used.

• Protein: Approximately 25-30 grams of protein per serving, making it a high-protein option.

• Carbohydrates: Approximately 15-20 grams of carbohydrates, mainly from the berries and yogurt.

• Fat: Approximately 5-7 grams of fat, primarily from almond milk and yogurt.

Health Benefits:

• The High-Protein Fruit Smoothie is an excellent option for those seeking to increase their protein intake while enjoying a delicious and satisfying drink. It's an ideal choice for individuals in the post-surgery phases, as it helps meet protein requirements while offering the benefits of antioxidants and essential nutrients from the mixed berries. The use of unsweetened ingredients aligns with dietary recommendations to limit added sugars. Additionally, the smoothie is easy to digest and provides hydration, making it an excellent option for those in recovery. It supports muscle preservation and healing while offering a tasty treat.

Creamy Tomato Soup

Ingredients:

• 2 cups of low-sodium tomato soup (store-bought or homemade)

• 1 scoop (approximately 10-15 grams) unflavored protein powder

• 1/2 cup of low-fat, unsweetened Greek yogurt

Step-by-Step Instructions:

1. In a medium-sized saucepan, pour in the low-sodium tomato soup. You can use your favorite store-bought brand or prepare homemade tomato soup with reduced salt.

2. Place the saucepan on the stove over medium heat. Heat the tomato soup until it's hot but not boiling. Stir occasionally to prevent sticking.

3. While the soup is heating, measure out one scoop of unflavored protein powder and set it aside.

4. Once the tomato soup is hot, reduce the heat to low to maintain a gentle simmer.

5. Slowly sprinkle the unflavored protein powder into the simmering tomato soup while continuously whisking to prevent any lumps from forming. Continue to whisk until the protein powder is fully dissolved.

6. After the protein powder has been fully incorporated,

add the low-fat, unsweetened Greek yogurt to the soup. Whisk it into the soup until the mixture becomes smooth and creamy.

7. Heat the soup for an additional 2-3 minutes, ensuring it's warmed through but not boiled.

8. Remove the saucepan from the heat.

9. Serve the Creamy Tomato Soup hot, and garnish with fresh herbs or a dollop of Greek yogurt if desired.

Portion Sizes:

• This recipe typically yields 2 servings of Creamy Tomato Soup. Each serving is approximately 1 cup.

Cooking Methods:

• The primary cooking method used in this recipe is stovetop heating, which allows for precise control over the heat to prevent boiling.

Storage and Reheating:

• Leftover soup can be stored in an airtight container in the refrigerator for 2-3 days. Reheat it gently on the stovetop over low heat, stirring occasionally to maintain the soup's creamy consistency.

Nutritional Information (per serving):

• Calories: Approximately 120-150 calories per serving, depending on the specific brand of tomato soup and protein powder used.

• Protein: Approximately 15-20 grams of protein per serving.

• Sodium: Less than 300 milligrams per serving with low-sodium tomato soup.

• Fat: Approximately 2-4 grams of fat, primarily from the yogurt.

Health Benefits:

• The Creamy Tomato Soup is designed to provide a satisfying and protein-rich meal, ideal for individuals in the post-surgery phases. It offers essential protein for healing and recovery while being gentle on the digestive system. The use of low-sodium tomato soup helps prevent excessive salt intake, and the addition of unflavored protein powder and Greek yogurt ensures the soup meets protein requirements. It's a creamy and flavorful option that supports hydration and provides a warm, comforting meal during the post-surgery journey.

Pureed Food Phase:

Protein-Packed Mashed Chicken

Ingredients:

• 1 cup of cooked, pureed chicken breast

• 1/2 cup of low-sodium chicken broth

• 1 scoop (approximately 10-15 grams) unflavored protein powder

Step-by-Step Instructions:

1. Begin by preparing the cooked, pureed chicken breast. You can cook the chicken breast by baking, boiling, or grilling until it's thoroughly cooked and then puree it in a blender or food processor until it reaches a smooth consistency.

2. In a saucepan, heat the low-sodium chicken broth over low to medium heat. Ensure that the broth is hot but not boiling.

3. While the broth is heating, measure out one scoop of unflavored protein powder and set it aside.

4. Once the broth is hot, slowly whisk the unflavored protein powder into the broth. Continue to whisk until the protein powder is fully dissolved.

5. Next, add the cooked, pureed chicken breast to the broth. Stir the mixture thoroughly to combine.

6. Continue to heat the mixture for an additional 2-3 minutes, ensuring it's heated through but not boiled.

7. Remove the saucepan from the heat.

8. Serve the Protein-Packed Mashed Chicken warm.

Portion Sizes:

• This recipe typically yields two servings of Protein-Packed Mashed Chicken. Each serving is approximately 1/2 cup.

Cooking Methods:

• The cooking method used in this recipe is stovetop heating to ensure precise control over the heat and prevent boiling.

Storage and Reheating:

• Any leftover Protein-Packed Mashed Chicken can be stored in an airtight container in the refrigerator for 2-3 days. Reheat it gently on the stovetop over low heat, stirring occasionally to maintain the dish's consistency.

Nutritional Information (per serving):

• Calories: Approximately 100-120 calories per serving, depending on the specific cooking method used for the chicken breast and the brand of protein powder.

• Protein: Approximately 15-20 grams of protein per

serving.

• Sodium: Less than 200 milligrams per serving with low-sodium chicken broth.

• Fat: Minimal to no fat content.

Health Benefits:

• Protein-Packed Mashed Chicken is tailored for individuals in the post-bariatric surgery phases, providing a substantial source of protein necessary for healing and muscle preservation. The recipe is gentle on the digestive system, offering a protein-rich and flavorful option. The use of low-sodium chicken broth helps control sodium intake, which is vital after bariatric surgery. Incorporating unflavored protein powder ensures the dish meets protein requirements, and it provides a comforting and easily digestible meal option during recovery.

Tofu and Veggie Puree

Ingredients:

• 1/2 cup of silken tofu

• 1/2 cup of cooked and pureed vegetables (e.g., carrots, peas)

• 1/4 cup of low-sodium vegetable broth

Step-by-Step Instructions:

1. Start by preparing the cooked and pureed vegetables. You can choose any soft, well-cooked vegetables that you prefer, such as carrots and peas. Cook them until they are tender, then puree them in a blender or food processor until they form a smooth consistency.

2. In a separate container, gently heat the low-sodium vegetable broth. Make sure it's hot but not boiling.

3. While the broth is heating, measure out the silken tofu and set it aside.

4. Once the broth is hot, place the silken tofu and pureed vegetables in a blender or food processor.

5. Slowly pour the hot vegetable broth into the blender or food processor.

6. Blend the mixture until it reaches a smooth and creamy consistency, ensuring that the tofu and vegetables are thoroughly incorporated into the broth.

7. Once the Tofu and Veggie Puree is well-blended, transfer it to a saucepan.

8. Heat the puree over low heat, stirring continuously for an additional 2-3 minutes to ensure it's warmed through.

9. Remove the saucepan from the heat.

10. Serve the Tofu and Veggie Puree warm.

Portion Sizes:

• This recipe typically yields one serving of Tofu and Veggie Puree, which is approximately 1 cup.

Cooking Methods:

• The primary cooking method used in this recipe is blending and stovetop heating to warm the puree.

Storage and Reheating:

• If you have any leftovers, you can store them in an airtight container in the refrigerator for 2-3 days. Reheat the puree gently on the stovetop over low heat, stirring occasionally to maintain its creamy consistency.

Nutritional Information (per serving):

• Calories: Approximately 150-200 calories per serving, depending on the specific vegetables used.

• Protein: Approximately 10-15 grams of protein per serving, mainly from silken tofu.

• Sodium: Less than 200 milligrams per serving with low-sodium vegetable broth.

• Fat: Approximately 5-7 grams of fat, primarily from silken tofu.

Health Benefits:

• Tofu and Veggie Puree is designed for individuals in the post-bariatric surgery phases, providing a nourishing and protein-rich option while maintaining a smooth texture that's easy to digest. Silken tofu serves as an excellent source of plant-based protein, while the pureed vegetables add essential nutrients and dietary fiber. The low-sodium vegetable broth helps control sodium intake, which is crucial after bariatric surgery. This puree offers a comforting and nutritious meal choice that supports healing and recovery. It also provides a source of plant-based protein for those with dietary preferences.

Soft Food Phase:

Scrambled Eggs with Spinach

Ingredients:

• 2 large scrambled eggs

• 1/4 cup of chopped fresh spinach

• 2 tablespoons of low-fat cottage cheese (optional)

Step-by-Step Instructions:

1. Begin by preparing the scrambled eggs. Crack two large eggs into a bowl, and whisk them until well beaten. You can add a pinch of salt and pepper for flavor, but be mindful of salt intake if you're using cottage cheese, which may already contain some sodium.

2. In a non-stick skillet over medium heat, add the beaten eggs. Cook the eggs, stirring gently and continuously until they are no longer runny but still moist. Be careful not to overcook them to maintain a tender texture.

3. As the eggs are nearly done, add the chopped fresh spinach to the skillet. Continue to cook and stir until the spinach wilts and the eggs are fully cooked.

4. If desired, fold in the low-fat cottage cheese into the scrambled eggs and spinach. This can add creaminess and additional protein to the dish.

5. Once everything is heated through and combined, transfer the Scrambled Eggs with Spinach to a plate.

6. Serve hot, and garnish with additional chopped fresh spinach or a sprinkle of cottage cheese if you prefer.

Portion Sizes:

• This recipe typically yields one serving of Scrambled Eggs with Spinach, which provides a satisfying meal.

Cooking Methods:

• The primary cooking method used in this recipe is stovetop cooking for the scrambled eggs. The spinach is added near the end of the cooking process.

Storage and Reheating:

• Scrambled Eggs with Spinach is best enjoyed freshly cooked. If you have any leftovers, they can be stored in an airtight container in the refrigerator for 1-2 days. Reheat gently in the microwave or on the stovetop, taking care not to overcook the eggs, as they can become rubbery with excessive reheating.

Nutritional Information (per serving):

• Calories: Approximately 200-250 calories per serving, depending on the addition of cottage cheese and cooking methods.

• Protein: Approximately 16-20 grams of protein per serving, which makes it a protein-rich meal.

• Fat: Approximately 10-12 grams of fat, primarily from the eggs and cottage cheese (if used).

• Carbohydrates: Minimal carbohydrates, primarily from the spinach.

Health Benefits:

• Scrambled Eggs with Spinach offers a protein-rich meal suitable for individuals in the post-bariatric surgery phases. Eggs are an excellent source of high-quality protein, while fresh spinach adds essential nutrients, fiber, and vitamins. The optional low-fat cottage cheese contributes additional protein and creaminess, making it a balanced and satisfying dish. It is easy to digest, provides important nutrients, and can be tailored to individual taste preferences. This recipe supports muscle preservation and healing during the post-surgery journey while delivering a tasty and nutritious meal.

Turkey and Mashed Potatoes

Ingredients:

• 4 ounces of lean ground turkey, cooked and finely diced

• 1/2 cup of mashed potatoes (without added butter)

• Low-sodium turkey gravy (in moderation)

Step-by-Step Instructions:

1. Begin by cooking the lean ground turkey. In a non-stick skillet over medium heat, cook the ground turkey until it's thoroughly done and slightly browned. You can season it with a pinch of salt and pepper, but go easy on the salt due to the use of gravy, which may contain sodium.

2. While the turkey is cooking, warm the mashed potatoes if they are not already hot. You can use a microwave or a stovetop pan for this.

3. Once the turkey is cooked and finely diced, place it on a plate.

4. In a separate container, heat the low-sodium turkey gravy. Be mindful of the portion size to keep the gravy's sodium content in check.

5. Serve the cooked and diced turkey alongside the mashed potatoes on a plate.

6. Pour a small amount of low-sodium turkey gravy over the turkey and potatoes. Use it in moderation to control sodium intake.

Portion Sizes:

• This recipe typically yields one serving of Turkey and Mashed Potatoes, providing a satisfying and well-portioned meal.

Cooking Methods:

• The primary cooking method used in this recipe is stovetop cooking for the ground turkey. The mashed potatoes are reheated as needed.

Storage and Reheating:

• It's recommended to prepare and consume this dish fresh. However, if you have leftovers, you can store them in separate airtight containers in the refrigerator for 1-2 days. Reheat gently in the microwave or on the stovetop, taking care not to overcook to prevent drying out the turkey.

Nutritional Information (per serving):

• Calories: Approximately 250-300 calories per serving, depending on the cooking method for the turkey and the portion size of gravy.

• Protein: Approximately 20-25 grams of protein per serving, making it a protein-rich meal.

• Fat: Approximately 5-7 grams of fat, primarily from the lean ground turkey.

• Carbohydrates: Approximately 20-25 grams of carbohydrates, mainly from the mashed potatoes.

Health Benefits:

• Turkey and Mashed Potatoes offer a balanced meal option with a substantial protein content, suitable for individuals in the post-bariatric surgery phases. Lean ground turkey provides high-quality protein, while mashed potatoes offer carbohydrates and comfort. Low-sodium turkey gravy should be used in moderation to control sodium intake. This meal is easy to digest and provides necessary nutrients while allowing for a familiar and satisfying dining experience. It supports muscle preservation and healing, making it a suitable option for those in recovery.

Transition to Regular Diet:

Grilled Salmon with Asparagus

Ingredients:

• 4-ounce grilled salmon fillet

• 1/2 cup of steamed asparagus spears

• Lemon juice and zest for flavor

Step-by-Step Instructions:

1. Begin by grilling the salmon fillet. You can season it with a touch of salt, pepper, and a drizzle of lemon juice for added flavor. Grill the salmon until it's cooked through and slightly charred, usually for about 4-5 minutes per side.

2. While the salmon is grilling, steam the asparagus spears. You can use a steamer or a microwave-safe container with a lid. Steam the asparagus until it's tender but still crisp, which typically takes 3-5 minutes.

3. Once the salmon is cooked, place it on a plate.

4. Arrange the steamed asparagus spears next to the salmon fillet.

5. Drizzle a little more lemon juice over both the salmon and asparagus for extra flavor.

6. Garnish with lemon zest for a fresh, citrusy aroma and taste.

Portion Sizes:

• This recipe typically yields one serving of Grilled Salmon with Asparagus, providing a well-balanced meal.

Cooking Methods:

• The primary cooking methods used in this recipe are grilling for the salmon and steaming for the asparagus.

Storage and Reheating:

• It's recommended to prepare and consume this dish fresh for the best flavor and texture. If you have leftovers, you can store the components separately in airtight containers in the refrigerator for up to 1-2 days. Reheat gently using a microwave or stovetop, being cautious not to overcook to maintain the salmon's tenderness.

Nutritional Information (per serving):

• Calories: Approximately 250-300 calories per serving, depending on the size of the salmon fillet.

• Protein: Approximately 25-30 grams of protein per serving, making it a high-protein meal.

• Fat: Approximately 10-12 grams of fat, primarily from the salmon.

• Carbohydrates: Approximately 10-15 grams of carbohydrates, mainly from the asparagus.

Health Benefits:

• Grilled Salmon with Asparagus is a nutritious and protein-rich meal suitable for individuals in the post-bariatric surgery phases. Salmon provides high-quality protein and healthy fats, while asparagus offers essential nutrients and dietary fiber. The use of lemon juice and zest adds a burst of fresh, citrusy flavor without the need for added sodium. This dish supports muscle preservation, healing, and overall health while providing a delicious and satisfying dining experience. It's easy to digest and packed with beneficial nutrients.

Quinoa and Black Bean Salad

Ingredients:

• 1 cup of cooked quinoa

• 1/2 cup of black beans, drained and rinsed

• 1/2 cup of diced bell peppers (choose your preferred color)

• 2 tablespoons of chopped cilantro

• Lime juice and olive oil dressing (mix 2 parts lime juice with 1 part olive oil)

Step-by-Step Instructions:

1. Start by cooking the quinoa according to the package instructions. Typically, it's cooked with a 2:1 ratio of water to quinoa. Allow it to cool before assembling the salad.

2. In a large mixing bowl, combine the cooked and cooled quinoa, drained and rinsed black beans, diced bell peppers, and chopped cilantro.

3. In a separate small bowl, prepare the lime juice and olive oil dressing by mixing two parts of lime juice with one part of olive oil. You can adjust the quantities to taste, and a pinch of salt and pepper can be added if desired, but go easy on the salt to control sodium intake.

4. Pour the lime juice and olive oil dressing over the quinoa,

beans, and vegetables.

5. Gently toss the salad to ensure that the dressing is evenly distributed and coats all the ingredients.

6. Allow the salad to marinate in the refrigerator for at least 30 minutes to let the flavors meld and intensify.

7. Serve the Quinoa and Black Bean Salad chilled, garnished with extra cilantro if desired.

Portion Sizes:

• This recipe typically yields 2-3 servings of Quinoa and Black Bean Salad, offering a satisfying portion for a meal.

Cooking Methods:

• The primary cooking method used in this recipe is boiling the quinoa. The rest of the ingredients are assembled without further cooking.

Storage and Reheating:

• This salad stores well in the refrigerator. You can keep any leftovers in an airtight container for up to 2-3 days. It is served chilled, so no reheating is necessary.

Nutritional Information (per serving):

• Calories: Approximately 250-300 calories per serving, depending on the portion size and dressing quantity.

• Protein: Approximately 8-10 grams of protein per serving.

• Fat: Approximately 5-7 grams of fat, mainly from the olive oil.

• Carbohydrates: Approximately 40-45 grams of carbohydrates, primarily from quinoa and vegetables.

Health Benefits:

• Quinoa and Black Bean Salad is a nutritious and balanced

meal suitable for individuals in the post-bariatric surgery phases. Quinoa is a complete protein source, and black beans add more protein and dietary fiber. Bell peppers contribute essential nutrients and a burst of color, while cilantro adds a fresh and vibrant flavor. The dressing with lime juice and olive oil is light and adds a delightful zing to the salad. It supports healing and recovery, offers beneficial nutrients, and is easy to digest, making it a healthy and delicious meal choice.

CHAPTER 4:

Low-Fat Recipes

Clear Liquid Phase:

Clear Chicken Broth with Herbs

Ingredients:

• 2 cups of low-sodium chicken broth

• Fresh herbs (e.g., parsley, thyme)

• Salt and pepper (in moderation)

Step-by-Step Instructions:

1. Pour the low-sodium chicken broth into a saucepan and place it over low to medium heat.

2. While the broth is heating, wash and chop a small handful of fresh herbs. You can use herbs like parsley and thyme for a flavorful addition to the broth.

3. Once the broth is hot but not boiling, add the fresh herbs to the saucepan. This will infuse the broth with a lovely herbal flavor.

4. Season the broth with a pinch of salt and a dash of pepper, being mindful of sodium intake. Remember that the broth is already low-sodium.

5. Allow the broth to simmer for 5-10 minutes to allow the herbs to infuse and the flavors to meld.

6. Remove the saucepan from heat and strain the clear chicken broth to remove the herbs and any solid particles.

7. Serve the Clear Chicken Broth with Herbs hot in a warm bowl.

Portion Sizes:

• This recipe typically yields one serving of Clear Chicken Broth with Herbs, providing a soothing and comforting portion.

Cooking Methods:

• The primary cooking method used in this recipe is stovetop heating and simmering to infuse the broth with herbs.

Storage and Reheating:

• Clear Chicken Broth with Herbs can be consumed immediately for the best flavor. However, if you have any leftovers, you can store them in an airtight container in the refrigerator for 1-2 days. Reheat gently on the stovetop or in the microwave.

Nutritional Information (per serving):

• Calories: Approximately 20-30 calories per serving, primarily from the chicken broth.

• Protein: Approximately 2-4 grams of protein per serving, depending on the broth's brand.

• Sodium: Less than 200 milligrams per serving with low-sodium chicken broth.

• Fat: Minimal to no fat content.

Health Benefits:

• Clear Chicken Broth with Herbs is a soothing and low-calorie option suitable for individuals in the post-bariatric surgery phases. It provides hydration and some protein from the chicken broth, while the fresh herbs add a delightful aroma and taste without significant calories or added sodium. The inclusion of herbs can also have potential health benefits, as they contain antioxidants and can contribute to a sense of comfort and well-being during the recovery process. It's gentle on the digestive system and can be a part of a liquid diet progression.

Iced Chamomile Tea

Ingredients:

• 2 chamomile tea bags

• Ice cubes

• Lemon wedge (optional)

Step-by-Step Instructions:

1. Boil water and pour it over the chamomile tea bags in a heatproof pitcher or container.

2. Allow the tea bags to steep in the hot water for about 5-7 minutes, or as per the recommended steeping time on the tea packaging. This will ensure that you get the full flavor and benefits of chamomile.

3. Once the tea has steeped, remove the tea bags and discard them.

4. Allow the chamomile tea to cool to room temperature, and then place it in the refrigerator to chill.

5. To serve, fill a glass with ice cubes.

6. Pour the chilled chamomile tea over the ice, leaving some room at the top of the glass.

7. If desired, squeeze a lemon wedge into the glass for added flavor and a touch of citrus.

8. Stir gently and serve the Iced Chamomile Tea cold.

Portion Sizes:

• This recipe typically yields one serving of Iced Chamomile Tea. Adjust the quantities based on your preferences.

Cooking Methods:

• The primary cooking method used in this recipe is tea steeping and cooling. No heating or cooking is involved.

Storage and Reheating:

• You can prepare and store the chamomile tea in the refrigerator for up to 2 days. However, it is best served fresh and chilled, so no reheating is necessary.

Nutritional Information (per serving):

• Calories: Approximately 0-5 calories per serving, as chamomile tea is naturally very low in calories.

• Carbohydrates: Minimal carbohydrates, primarily from the chamomile tea.

Health Benefits:

• Iced Chamomile Tea is a soothing and refreshing beverage with potential health benefits. Chamomile is known for its calming and anti-inflammatory properties, which can be especially beneficial during the post-bariatric surgery journey. It can aid in digestion and relaxation. The addition of a lemon wedge provides a hint of citrus flavor and vitamin C. This tea is also naturally caffeine-free and low in calories, making it a hydrating and gentle option for those in recovery. It can help reduce inflammation and promote a sense of well-being.

Full Liquid Phase:

Creamy Low-Fat Yogurt Smoothie

Ingredients:

• 1 cup of low-fat plain yogurt

• 1/2 cup of frozen mixed berries

• 1 scoop (approximately 10-15 grams) unflavored protein powder

• 1/2 cup of unsweetened almond milk

Step-by-Step Instructions:

1. In a blender, combine the low-fat plain yogurt, frozen mixed berries, unflavored protein powder, and unsweetened almond milk.

2. Blend the ingredients until they form a smooth and creamy consistency. You can adjust the amount of almond milk to achieve your desired thickness.

3. Taste the smoothie and add a bit of honey or a natural sweetener if needed. Be mindful of the sugar content if you choose to sweeten it.

4. Pour the Creamy Low-Fat Yogurt Smoothie into a glass.

5. Serve the smoothie chilled, and you can garnish it with additional berries or a sprig of mint if desired.

Portion Sizes:

• This recipe typically yields one serving of Creamy Low-Fat Yogurt Smoothie, providing a satisfying and well-portioned meal or snack.

Preparation and Cooking Methods:

• The primary method for this recipe is blending to create a smooth and creamy texture.

Storage and Reheating:

• The Creamy Low-Fat Yogurt Smoothie is best enjoyed freshly made. However, if you have leftovers, you can store them in a covered container in the refrigerator for up to 24 hours. Be sure to give it a good stir before consuming any leftovers, as separation may occur. Avoid freezing, as it can alter the texture.

Nutritional Information (per serving):

• Calories: Approximately 250-300 calories per serving, depending on the specific ingredients and sweeteners used.

• Protein: Approximately 15-20 grams of protein per serving, mainly from the yogurt and protein powder.

• Fat: Approximately 5-7 grams of fat, primarily from the yogurt.

• Carbohydrates: Approximately 20-25 grams of carbohydrates, mainly from the berries and almond milk.

Health Benefits:

• The Creamy Low-Fat Yogurt Smoothie is a nutritious and protein-rich option, ideal for individuals in the post-bariatric surgery phases. Low-fat yogurt provides high-quality protein and calcium, while frozen mixed berries contribute essential nutrients, antioxidants, and natural sweetness. Unflavored protein powder enhances the protein content for healing and muscle preservation. Unsweetened almond milk offers creaminess without excess sugar. This smoothie supports recovery and overall health, making it a delightful and satisfying choice for a meal or snack. It is easy to digest and can be tailored to individual preferences and dietary needs.

Low-Fat Cream of Broccoli Soup

Ingredients:

• 2 cups of steamed broccoli

• 1/2 cup of low-fat Greek yogurt

• 2 cups of low-sodium vegetable broth

Step-by-Step Instructions:

1. Begin by steaming the broccoli until it's tender but still bright green. This can be done using a steamer or by microwaving it with a little water for about 3-5 minutes.

2. Once the broccoli is steamed, transfer it to a blender or food processor.

3. Add the low-fat Greek yogurt and low-sodium vegetable broth to the blender with the steamed broccoli.

4. Blend the mixture until it forms a smooth and creamy consistency. If the soup is too thick, you can add a bit more vegetable broth until you reach your desired thickness.

5. Pour the Low-Fat Cream of Broccoli Soup into a saucepan and gently heat it over low to medium heat. Stir occasionally until it's warmed through, but do not allow it to boil.

6. Once the soup is heated, pour it into a bowl.

7. You can garnish the soup with a few steamed broccoli florets or a dollop of Greek yogurt for added visual appeal.

8. Serve the Low-Fat Cream of Broccoli Soup hot and enjoy.

Portion Sizes:

• This recipe typically yields 2-3 servings of Low-Fat Cream of Broccoli Soup, offering a satisfying and nutritious meal.

Cooking Methods:

• The primary cooking methods used in this recipe are steaming the broccoli and blending to create a smooth soup. A final heating step is performed on the stovetop.

Storage and Reheating:

• Low-Fat Cream of Broccoli Soup can be prepared ahead and stored in an airtight container in the refrigerator for up to 2-3 days. Reheat gently on the stovetop, stirring occasionally to maintain the creamy consistency.

Nutritional Information (per serving):

• Calories: Approximately 100-150 calories per serving, depending on portion size and yogurt quantity.

• Protein: Approximately 7-10 grams of protein per serving, mainly from the Greek yogurt.

• Fat: Approximately 3-5 grams of fat, primarily from the Greek yogurt.

• Carbohydrates: Approximately 10-15 grams of carbohydrates, mainly from the broccoli.

Health Benefits:

• Low-Fat Cream of Broccoli Soup is a nutritious and protein-rich option suitable for individuals in the post-bariatric surgery phases. Broccoli provides essential nutrients and dietary fiber, while low-fat Greek yogurt offers high-quality protein and creaminess without excess fat. The low-sodium vegetable broth adds flavor without an excess of salt. This soup supports recovery and overall health, making it a satisfying choice for a meal. It is easy to digest and can be tailored to individual preferences and dietary needs. The combination of nutrients promotes healing and muscle preservation.

Pureed Food Phase:

Low-Fat Chicken and Vegetable Puree

Ingredients:

• 1 cup of cooked, pureed chicken breast

• 1 cup of pureed cooked vegetables (e.g., carrots, zucchini)

• 1 cup of low-sodium chicken broth

• Fresh herbs for flavor (e.g., parsley, thyme)

Step-by-Step Instructions:

1. Start by cooking the chicken breast. You can simmer it in water until it's thoroughly cooked. Then, puree the cooked chicken breast in a food processor or blender until you achieve a smooth consistency.

2. In a separate pot, steam or cook the vegetables until they are tender. This can be done with carrots, zucchini, or any preferred vegetables. Puree the cooked vegetables to a smooth consistency.

3. Combine the pureed chicken breast and pureed vegetables in a saucepan.

4. Add the low-sodium chicken broth to the mixture, adjusting the quantity to achieve your preferred

consistency.

5. Place the saucepan over low to medium heat and gently heat the mixture. Stir occasionally until it's warmed through but do not allow it to boil.

6. Season with fresh herbs like parsley or thyme for added flavor. Herbs can also add potential health benefits.

7. Serve the Low-Fat Chicken and Vegetable Puree hot in a bowl.

Portion Sizes:

• This recipe typically yields 2-3 servings of Low-Fat Chicken and Vegetable Puree, providing a satisfying and nutrient-rich meal.

Cooking Methods:

• The primary cooking methods used in this recipe are boiling the chicken breast, steaming or boiling the vegetables, and gently heating the puree on the stovetop.

Storage and Reheating:

• Low-Fat Chicken and Vegetable Puree can be prepared ahead and stored in the refrigerator in an airtight container for up to 2-3 days. Reheat gently on the stovetop, adding a bit of water or broth if needed to adjust the consistency.

Nutritional Information (per serving):

• Calories: Approximately 100-150 calories per serving, depending on the portion size and broth quantity.

• Protein: Approximately 15-20 grams of protein per serving, primarily from the chicken breast.

• Fat: Minimal to low fat content, mainly from the chicken.

• Carbohydrates: Approximately 5-10 grams of carbohydrates, primarily from the vegetables.

Health Benefits:

• Low-Fat Chicken and Vegetable Puree is a nutritious and protein-rich option suitable for individuals in the post-bariatric surgery phases. It provides a combination of lean protein from the chicken and essential nutrients from the vegetables. The use of low-sodium chicken broth adds flavor without excessive salt. The inclusion of fresh herbs not only enhances the taste but also contributes to potential health benefits, such as antioxidants and digestive support. This puree is gentle on the digestive system, easy to digest, and supports healing and overall health during the recovery process.

Mashed Sweet Potatoes

Ingredients:

• 1 cup of cooked, mashed sweet potatoes (without added butter)

• 2 tablespoons of low-fat plain yogurt

• 1/4 teaspoon of ground cinnamon

Step-by-Step Instructions:

1. Begin by cooking the sweet potatoes until they are tender. You can do this by boiling, steaming, or baking them in the oven. Once cooked, allow them to cool slightly.

2. Place the cooked sweet potatoes in a mixing bowl.

3. Add the low-fat plain yogurt and ground cinnamon to the bowl.

4. Use a fork or a potato masher to mash and mix the ingredients together until you achieve a smooth and creamy consistency.

5. If the mixture seems too dry, you can add a bit more yogurt until you reach your desired texture.

6. Taste the mashed sweet potatoes and adjust the amount of cinnamon or yogurt if needed.

7. Serve the Mashed Sweet Potatoes as a side dish. You can garnish with a sprinkle of additional ground cinnamon for extra flavor and visual appeal.

Portion Sizes:

• This recipe typically yields 2-3 servings of Mashed Sweet Potatoes, providing a delicious and satisfying side dish.

Cooking Methods:

• The primary cooking method used in this recipe is cooking the sweet potatoes, followed by mashing and mixing.

Storage and Reheating:

• Mashed Sweet Potatoes can be prepared ahead and stored in the refrigerator in an airtight container for up to 2-3 days. Reheat gently in the microwave or on the stovetop, adding a bit of water or yogurt if needed to adjust the consistency.

Nutritional Information (per serving):

• Calories: Approximately 100-150 calories per serving, depending on portion size and yogurt quantity.

• Protein: Approximately 2-4 grams of protein per serving, mainly from the yogurt.

• Fat: Minimal to low fat content, mainly from the yogurt.

• Carbohydrates: Approximately 20-25 grams of carbohydrates, mainly from the sweet potatoes.

Health Benefits:

• Mashed Sweet Potatoes are a nutritious and fiber-rich side dish suitable for individuals in the post-bariatric surgery phases. Sweet potatoes are an excellent source of complex carbohydrates, vitamins, and dietary fiber. The use of low-fat plain yogurt adds creaminess and a bit of protein without excessive fat. Ground cinnamon not only enhances the flavor but may also have potential health benefits, such as anti-inflammatory properties. This dish supports overall health and digestive comfort, making it a wholesome and tasty addition to your post-surgery diet.

Soft Food Phase:

Baked Cod with Lemon and Herbs

Ingredients:

• 1 cod fillet (approximately 4-6 oz)

• Juice and zest of 1 lemon

• Fresh herbs (e.g., dill, parsley)

• Salt and pepper to taste

Step-by-Step Instructions:

1. Preheat your oven to 375°F (190°C) to prepare for baking.

2. Place the cod fillet on a baking sheet lined with parchment paper or lightly greased to prevent sticking.

3. Squeeze the juice from the lemon over the cod fillet. The lemon juice will infuse the fish with a bright, fresh flavor.

4. Grate the zest from the lemon using a fine grater or

zester and sprinkle it over the cod. Lemon zest adds an extra layer of citrusy aroma and taste.

5. Season the cod fillet with salt and pepper to taste.

6. Choose your preferred fresh herbs, such as dill, parsley, or a combination of both. Chop the herbs finely and sprinkle them over the cod fillet.

7. Bake the cod in the preheated oven for about 15-20 minutes or until it's cooked through and flakes easily with a fork. Cooking times may vary depending on the thickness of the fillet, so keep an eye on it.

8. Once the cod is cooked, remove it from the oven and serve immediately.

Portion Sizes:

• This recipe typically yields one serving of Baked Cod with Lemon and Herbs. Adjust the quantities based on your preferences.

Cooking Methods:

• The primary cooking method used in this recipe is baking, which helps retain the fish's moisture and flavor.

Storage and Reheating:

• Baked Cod with Lemon and Herbs is best enjoyed fresh and right out of the oven. However, if you have leftovers, store them in an airtight container in the refrigerator for up to 2 days. To reheat, place the cod on a microwave-safe plate, cover with a microwave-safe lid or plastic wrap, and reheat gently in the microwave for short intervals, checking frequently to avoid overcooking.

Nutritional Information (per serving):

• Calories: Approximately 150-200 calories per serving,

depending on the size of the cod fillet.

• Protein: Approximately 25-30 grams of protein per serving, mainly from the cod.

• Fat: Minimal fat content, primarily from the fish.

• Carbohydrates: Approximately 2-4 grams of carbohydrates, primarily from the lemon zest.

Health Benefits:

• Baked Cod with Lemon and Herbs is a nutritious and protein-packed dish suitable for individuals in the post-bariatric surgery phases. Cod is a lean source of protein and provides essential nutrients, while lemon and fresh herbs add a burst of flavor and potential health benefits. The lemon's acidity can aid in digestion, and the herbs contribute antioxidants and freshness. This dish is gentle on the digestive system, easy to digest, and supports recovery and overall health during the post-surgery journey.

Low-Fat Turkey and Rice Soup

Ingredients:

• 4 oz of lean ground turkey

• 1/2 cup of cooked rice

• 2 cups of low-sodium chicken broth

• 1/2 cup of chopped carrots

• 1/2 cup of chopped celery

Step-by-Step Instructions:

1. In a soup pot or a saucepan, place the lean ground turkey over medium heat. Break the turkey into small pieces with a spatula as it cooks.

2. Continue cooking the turkey until it's browned and cooked through. Drain any excess fat, if needed.

3. Add the chopped carrots and celery to the pot with the turkey. Sauté them for a few minutes until they begin to soften.

4. Pour in the low-sodium chicken broth and bring the mixture to a gentle simmer. Allow it to simmer for about 15-20 minutes, or until the vegetables are tender.

5. Stir in the cooked rice and allow the soup to simmer for an additional 5 minutes to heat the rice.

6. Taste the soup and adjust the seasoning with salt and pepper, if desired. Be mindful of the salt content, as low-sodium broth is used.

7. Once the soup is heated through and the flavors meld, remove it from heat.

8. Serve the Low-Fat Turkey and Rice Soup hot in bowls.

Portion Sizes:

• This recipe typically yields 2-3 servings of Low-Fat Turkey and Rice Soup, providing a filling and nutrient-rich meal.

Cooking Methods:

• The primary cooking method used in this recipe is sautéing, simmering, and gentle heating on the stovetop.

Storage and Reheating:

• Low-Fat Turkey and Rice Soup can be prepared ahead and

stored in the refrigerator in an airtight container for up to 2-3 days. Reheat on the stovetop, adding a bit of water or additional broth if needed to adjust the consistency.

Nutritional Information (per serving):

• Calories: Approximately 150-200 calories per serving, depending on portion size.

• Protein: Approximately 15-20 grams of protein per serving, primarily from the turkey.

• Fat: Minimal fat content, mainly from the turkey.

• Carbohydrates: Approximately 15-20 grams of carbohydrates, primarily from the rice and vegetables.

Health Benefits:

• Low-Fat Turkey and Rice Soup is a hearty and protein-rich option suitable for individuals in the post-bariatric surgery phases. Lean ground turkey provides high-quality protein without excessive fat, while cooked rice adds comforting carbohydrates. The inclusion of chopped carrots and celery offers essential nutrients and dietary fiber. Low-sodium chicken broth provides flavor without an excess of salt. This soup is gentle on the digestive system, easy to digest, and supports recovery and overall health during the post-surgery journey. It provides a well-balanced meal option with essential nutrients.

Transition to Regular Diet:

Grilled Chicken Breast with Steamed Vegetables

Ingredients:

• 4 oz of grilled chicken breast

• Steamed broccoli, carrots, and cauliflower (approximately

1/2 cup of each)

• Lemon juice for flavor

Step-by-Step Instructions:

1. Start by grilling the chicken breast. You can season it with a little salt, pepper, and any preferred herbs or spices before grilling.

2. While the chicken is grilling, prepare the steamed vegetables. You can steam them on the stovetop or in a microwave-safe steamer. Steam until they are tender but still crisp, which usually takes about 5-7 minutes.

3. Once the chicken breast is cooked and the vegetables are steamed, remove them from their respective cooking methods.

4. Squeeze fresh lemon juice over the grilled chicken breast for added flavor. Lemon juice also adds a zesty freshness to the dish.

5. Arrange the steamed vegetables alongside the grilled chicken breast on a plate.

6. Serve the Grilled Chicken Breast with Steamed Vegetables hot, and you can drizzle a bit more lemon juice over the vegetables if desired.

Portion Sizes:

• This recipe typically yields one serving of Grilled Chicken Breast with Steamed Vegetables, providing a nutritious and well-balanced meal.

Cooking Methods:

• The primary cooking methods used in this recipe are grilling the chicken and steaming the vegetables.

Storage and Reheating:

• Grilled Chicken Breast with Steamed Vegetables is best enjoyed freshly made. However, if you have leftovers, you can store the grilled chicken and steamed vegetables in separate airtight containers in the refrigerator for up to 2 days. Reheat gently on the stovetop or in the microwave, adding a touch of water to the vegetables if needed to maintain their tenderness.

Nutritional Information (per serving):

• Calories: Approximately 150-200 calories per serving, depending on portion size.

• Protein: Approximately 25-30 grams of protein per serving, primarily from the chicken.

• Fat: Minimal fat content, mainly from the chicken.

• Carbohydrates: Approximately 5-10 grams of carbohydrates, primarily from the steamed vegetables.

Health Benefits:

• Grilled Chicken Breast with Steamed Vegetables is a highly nutritious and protein-rich dish suitable for individuals in the post-bariatric surgery phases. The lean grilled chicken breast provides essential protein without excessive fat, while the steamed vegetables offer a variety of vitamins and dietary fiber. Lemon juice adds flavor and freshness and may aid in digestion. This dish is gentle on the digestive system, easy to digest, and supports recovery and overall health during the post-surgery journey. It provides a well-balanced meal with essential nutrients for healing and muscle preservation.

Quinoa and Black Bean Salad with Lime Vinaigrette

Ingredients:

- 1/2 cup of cooked quinoa

- 1/2 cup of black beans, drained and rinsed

- 1/2 cup of chopped bell peppers (red, yellow, or green)

- Lime vinaigrette (made with lime juice and minimal oil)

Step-by-Step Instructions:

1. Start by cooking quinoa according to the package instructions. Typically, you'll use 1 cup of water for 1/2 cup of quinoa. Bring to a boil, then simmer for about 15 minutes, or until the quinoa is fluffy and the water is absorbed. Once cooked, let it cool.

2. In a mixing bowl, combine the cooked and cooled quinoa, drained and rinsed black beans, and the chopped bell peppers. You can use a variety of colors for a visually appealing salad.

3. Prepare the lime vinaigrette. Squeeze fresh lime juice into a separate bowl and add a minimal amount of oil (e.g., olive oil or a heart-healthy oil of your choice). Whisk these ingredients together. You can add a touch of salt and pepper for flavor, if desired.

4. Pour the lime vinaigrette over the quinoa, black beans, and bell peppers. Toss the salad gently to coat all the ingredients evenly with the vinaigrette.

5. Taste the salad and adjust the seasoning or add more vinaigrette if needed.

6. Serve the Quinoa and Black Bean Salad with Lime Vinaigrette immediately or refrigerate it for a chilled salad.

Portion Sizes:

- This recipe typically yields 1-2 servings of Quinoa and

Black Bean Salad, providing a refreshing and nutrient-rich side or main dish.

Cooking Methods:

• The primary cooking method used in this recipe is cooking quinoa, followed by mixing and tossing the ingredients to prepare the salad.

Storage and Reheating:

• Quinoa and Black Bean Salad with Lime Vinaigrette can be stored in the refrigerator in an airtight container for up to 2 days. It's suitable for serving chilled. If you prefer to reheat it slightly, you can do so in the microwave for a short time, but this dish is generally enjoyed cold.

Nutritional Information (per serving):

• Calories: Approximately 200-250 calories per serving, depending on portion size and the amount of vinaigrette used.

• Protein: Approximately 6-8 grams of protein per serving, primarily from quinoa and black beans.

• Fat: Minimal fat content, mainly from the vinaigrette.

• Carbohydrates: Approximately 40-50 grams of carbohydrates, primarily from quinoa and vegetables.

Health Benefits:

• Quinoa and Black Bean Salad with Lime Vinaigrette is a nutritious and fiber-rich dish suitable for individuals in the post-bariatric surgery phases. Quinoa is a protein-rich and gluten-free grain, while black beans offer additional protein and dietary fiber. The inclusion of bell peppers adds vitamins and visual appeal. Lime vinaigrette provides a zesty and refreshing flavor without an excessive amount of oil, making this salad a healthy and satisfying choice. It supports recovery and overall health by providing essential nutrients and promoting digestive comfort.

CHAPTER 5:

Low-Sugar Recipes

Clear Liquid Phase:

Sugar-Free Jello

Ingredients:

• 1 packet of sugar-free gelatin (any flavor of your choice)

• 1 cup of boiling water

Step-by-Step Instructions:

1. In a heatproof mixing bowl, empty the contents of the sugar-free gelatin packet.

2. Boil 1 cup of water, and carefully pour the boiling water over the gelatin powder in the bowl.

3. Stir the mixture thoroughly with a spoon until the gelatin is completely dissolved.

4. Allow the mixture to cool for a few minutes.

5. Once the mixture has cooled slightly, pour it into individual serving cups or molds. You can use silicone molds or small dessert cups.

6. Place the cups or molds in the refrigerator to set. It typically takes about 2-4 hours for the Jello to firm up, but it's best to leave it in the fridge for a longer period for a better texture.

7. Once the Sugar-Free Jello has set, it's ready to be served. You can enjoy it straight from the cups or molds.

Portion Sizes:

• The number of servings depends on the size of your individual cups or molds. This recipe makes enough to fill approximately 4 standard dessert cups.

Cooking Methods:

• The primary method in this recipe is dissolving the gelatin in boiling water and allowing it to set in the refrigerator.

Storage and Reheating:

• Sugar-Free Jello can be stored in the refrigerator for up to 2-3 days in an airtight container. Reheating is not necessary for Jello, as it is typically served chilled.

Nutritional Information (per serving):

• Calories: Approximately 5-10 calories per serving, depending on the specific brand of sugar-free gelatin used and portion size.

• Protein: Minimal protein content.

• Fat: Minimal fat content.

• Carbohydrates: Approximately 0-1 gram of carbohydrates per serving.

Health Benefits:

• Sugar-Free Jello is a low-calorie and sugar-free dessert option suitable for individuals in the post-bariatric surgery phases. It provides a sweet and satisfying treat without added sugars, making it a suitable choice for those looking to manage their sugar intake. While it doesn't offer significant nutritional content, it can be a pleasant and guilt-free way to satisfy a sweet craving. Additionally, Jello is easy to digest and gentle on the stomach, making it a good option for individuals in the early stages of their post-surgery diet.

Mint-Infused Water

Ingredients:

• Fresh mint leaves

• Water

• Optional: a splash of lemon or lime juice

Step-by-Step Instructions:

1. Begin by thoroughly rinsing the fresh mint leaves under cold running water. This step helps remove any impurities or debris from the leaves.

2. In a pitcher or a large glass, place a handful of fresh mint leaves. You can adjust the quantity based on your preference for mint flavor.

3. Pour cool or room temperature water over the mint leaves in the pitcher or glass. The amount of water depends on how concentrated you want the flavor. A standard ratio is approximately 8-10 cups of water for every handful of mint leaves.

4. If you'd like a hint of citrus flavor, add a splash of fresh lemon or lime juice to the infused water.

5. Stir the water gently to help release the mint flavor and allow it to infuse. You can use a long spoon for this purpose.

6. Let the Mint-Infused Water sit at room temperature or in

the refrigerator for at least 1-2 hours, but longer infusion time yields a stronger flavor.

7. Before serving, you can strain the water to remove the mint leaves if you prefer, but it's not necessary.

8. Serve the Mint-Infused Water in glasses with ice cubes and garnish with a fresh mint sprig, if desired. Enjoy the refreshing drink.

Portion Sizes:

• The number of servings depends on the amount of water and mint leaves used. A standard batch can make approximately 8-10 servings.

Preparation and Cooking Methods:

• Mint-Infused Water does not involve cooking. It is made through the process of infusion, allowing the mint leaves to flavor the water naturally.

Storage and Reheating:

• Mint-Infused Water can be stored in the refrigerator for up to 2 days. It's best when served freshly made. No reheating is required.

Nutritional Information (per serving):

• Calories: Almost negligible (usually less than 5 calories per serving).

• Protein: Minimal to no protein content.

• Fat: No fat content.

• Carbohydrates: Minimal carbohydrates, primarily from the mint leaves.

Health Benefits:

• Mint-Infused Water is a hydrating and refreshing

beverage option suitable for individuals in the post-bariatric surgery phases. Mint leaves add a pleasant, natural flavor without the need for added sugars or artificial sweeteners. Mint may also help soothe the digestive system. The optional addition of lemon or lime juice provides a touch of vitamin C and a citrusy twist. This infused water is calorie-friendly, encourages hydration, and supports overall health during the post-surgery journey. It's an excellent alternative to sugary beverages and a great way to enjoy the taste of mint.

Full Liquid Phase:

Berry Protein Smoothie

Ingredients:

• 1 scoop of unflavored protein powder

• 1/2 cup of frozen mixed berries (blueberries, strawberries, raspberries, etc.)

• 1 cup of unsweetened almond milk

• Stevia or another sugar substitute (optional)

Step-by-Step Instructions:

1. In a blender, add the unflavored protein powder, frozen mixed berries, and unsweetened almond milk.

2. If you prefer a sweeter taste, you can add Stevia or another sugar substitute to the blender. The amount can vary depending on your taste preferences, so start with a small amount and adjust as needed.

3. Blend the ingredients on high speed until you achieve a smooth and creamy consistency. This usually takes about 30 seconds to 1 minute.

4. Stop the blender and check the taste. If necessary, you can add more sugar substitute or adjust the thickness by adding more almond milk.

5. Once the smoothie reaches your desired taste and consistency, pour it into a glass.

6. Serve the Berry Protein Smoothie immediately. You can also add a few additional berries or a mint sprig as garnish if desired.

Portion Sizes:

• This recipe typically yields one serving of Berry Protein Smoothie, providing a filling and nutritious drink.

Preparation and Cooking Methods:

• The primary method in this recipe is blending the ingredients to create a smooth and creamy smoothie.

Storage and Reheating:

• Berry Protein Smoothie is best enjoyed freshly made to preserve its texture and freshness. However, if you have leftovers, you can store them in the refrigerator for a short time, but keep in mind that the texture may change when stored. Reblend the smoothie before consuming any leftovers. Reheating is not necessary, as this smoothie is typically served cold.

Nutritional Information (per serving):

• Calories: Approximately 200-250 calories per serving, depending on the specific brand of protein powder and the amount of sugar substitute used.

• Protein: Approximately 20-25 grams of protein per serving, primarily from the protein powder.

• Fat: Minimal fat content, mainly from almond milk.

• Carbohydrates: Approximately 15-20 grams of carbohydrates, primarily from the berries and almond milk.

Health Benefits:

• The Berry Protein Smoothie is a high-protein, low-sugar, and fiber-rich option suitable for individuals in the post-bariatric surgery phases. The unflavored protein powder provides essential protein without excessive added sugar, while the frozen mixed berries offer antioxidants and natural sweetness. Unsweetened almond milk keeps the smoothie light on calories and fat. The optional sugar substitute allows for customization without using refined sugars. This smoothie is gentle on the digestive system, easy to digest, and supports recovery and overall health during the post-surgery journey. It's a satisfying way to meet protein needs and enjoy the flavors of mixed berries without added sugars.

Low-Sugar Chai Latte

Ingredients:

• Unsweetened chai tea (tea bags or concentrate)

• Unsweetened almond milk

• Sugar substitute (e.g., stevia or monk fruit)

Step-by-Step Instructions:

1. Start by brewing a cup of unsweetened chai tea using tea bags or concentrate, following the package instructions.

Ensure that no sugar or sweeteners are added during the brewing process.

2. While the tea is brewing, heat 1 cup of unsweetened almond milk in a saucepan on the stovetop. Heat it over low to medium heat, making sure not to bring it to a boil. Heat until it's warm and steaming.

3. Once the chai tea is ready, remove the tea bag or concentrate and discard it.

4. In a cup, mix the warm unsweetened chai tea and the steaming unsweetened almond milk. You can adjust the ratio to your taste preference, but a 1:1 ratio is a good starting point.

5. Add the sugar substitute of your choice to the chai latte. The amount depends on your sweetness preference, so start with a small amount and adjust as needed.

6. Stir the chai latte to dissolve the sugar substitute, making sure it's well incorporated.

7. Taste the chai latte and add more sugar substitute if desired.

8. Serve the Low-Sugar Chai Latte hot and enjoy.

Portion Sizes:

• This recipe typically yields one serving of Low-Sugar Chai Latte, providing a comforting and low-sugar drink.

Cooking Methods:

• The primary cooking method in this recipe is brewing chai tea and heating almond milk, followed by mixing the ingredients to create the latte.

Storage and Reheating:

• Low-Sugar Chai Latte is best enjoyed freshly made to

preserve its warmth and flavor. Reheating can be done on the stovetop or in the microwave if you have leftover chai latte, but do not bring it to a boil.

Nutritional Information (per serving):

• Calories: Approximately 30-40 calories per serving, depending on the specific brand of almond milk and the amount of sugar substitute used.

• Protein: Minimal protein content, primarily from almond milk.

• Fat: Minimal fat content, mainly from almond milk.

• Carbohydrates: Approximately 5-10 grams of carbohydrates, primarily from almond milk.

Health Benefits:

• The Low-Sugar Chai Latte is a comforting and low-sugar beverage suitable for individuals in the post-bariatric surgery phases. Unsweetened chai tea provides flavor and spices without added sugars, while unsweetened almond milk offers a dairy-free and low-calorie base. The sugar substitute allows for customization without using refined sugars. This latte is gentle on the digestive system, easy to digest, and supports recovery and overall health during the post-surgery journey. It's a warm and soothing way to enjoy the flavors of chai without excess sugar.

Pureed Food Phase:

Applesauce with Cinnamon

Ingredients:

• Unsweetened applesauce

• Ground cinnamon

• Stevia or another sugar substitute (optional)

Step-by-Step Instructions:

1. Measure the desired amount of unsweetened applesauce and place it in a bowl. The amount will depend on how many servings you want to prepare.

2. Sprinkle ground cinnamon over the unsweetened applesauce. The quantity of cinnamon depends on your taste preference, but start with a small amount and adjust as needed. Cinnamon adds a warm and fragrant flavor to the applesauce.

3. If you prefer a sweeter taste, you can add Stevia or another sugar substitute to the applesauce. Adjust the amount based on your desired level of sweetness.

4. Stir the ingredients in the bowl thoroughly to evenly distribute the cinnamon and sweetener, if used.

5. Taste the Applesauce with Cinnamon and adjust the cinnamon and sweetness to your liking.

6. Serve the applesauce as a side dish or snack, and enjoy its comforting flavors.

Portion Sizes:

• The number of servings depends on the amount of unsweetened applesauce you use. This recipe is flexible and can be made in small or large quantities.

Preparation Methods:

• Applesauce with Cinnamon is a no-cook recipe that requires mixing and stirring.

Storage and Reheating:

• Applesauce with Cinnamon can be stored in the refrigerator for several days. There is no need for reheating, as it's typically served cold.

Nutritional Information (per serving):

• Calories: Approximately 20-30 calories per serving, depending on the portion size and the use of sugar substitute.

• Protein: Minimal protein content.

• Fat: Minimal fat content.

• Carbohydrates: Approximately 5-10 grams of carbohydrates, primarily from the applesauce.

Health Benefits:

• Applesauce with Cinnamon is a low-calorie and naturally sweet snack suitable for individuals in the post-bariatric surgery phases. Unsweetened applesauce provides fiber, vitamins, and minerals without added sugars, while ground cinnamon adds flavor and a hint of warmth. The optional sugar substitute allows for customization without using refined sugars. This snack is easy to digest and gentle on the digestive system, making it a convenient choice for those in the early stages of their post-surgery diet. It supports recovery and overall health by providing essential nutrients and a satisfying taste.

Vanilla Protein Pudding

Ingredients:

• Sugar-free vanilla pudding mix

• Unflavored protein powder

• Skim milk or a milk alternative

Step-by-Step Instructions:

1. In a mixing bowl, combine the sugar-free vanilla pudding mix and unflavored protein powder.

2. Gradually add skim milk or a milk alternative to the dry ingredients while whisking continuously. The amount of milk added should align with the instructions on the pudding mix package. Follow the package's guidelines for the best results.

3. Whisk the mixture thoroughly to ensure the pudding mix and protein powder are fully dissolved into the milk. This may take a couple of minutes.

4. Once the mixture is smooth, transfer it to a saucepan.

5. Heat the mixture over low to medium heat while stirring continuously. Bring it to a gentle simmer and let it simmer for 2-3 minutes. This helps thicken the pudding and ensures that the protein powder is fully incorporated.

6. Remove the saucepan from the heat and let the pudding cool for a few minutes.

7. Pour the warm pudding into serving dishes or ramekins.

8. Let the Vanilla Protein Pudding cool to room temperature, and then refrigerate it for a few hours or until it's fully set.

9. Once the pudding has set, it's ready to be served.

Portion Sizes:

• The number of servings depends on the portion size and the amount of pudding prepared. This recipe can typically yield 4-6 servings.

Cooking Methods:

• The main cooking method in this recipe involves mixing, heating, and cooling to set the pudding.

Storage and Reheating:

• Store any leftover Vanilla Protein Pudding in the refrigerator. It can be reheated on the stovetop if desired, but it's typically served cold.

Nutritional Information (per serving):

• Calories: Approximately 70-100 calories per serving, depending on the specific brand of pudding mix, protein powder, and milk used.

• Protein: Approximately 8-10 grams of protein per serving, primarily from the protein powder.

• Fat: Minimal fat content, mainly from the milk.

• Carbohydrates: Approximately 5-10 grams of carbohydrates, primarily from the pudding mix.

Health Benefits:

• Vanilla Protein Pudding is a satisfying and protein-rich dessert suitable for individuals in the post-bariatric surgery phases. The combination of sugar-free vanilla pudding mix and unflavored protein powder offers a delightful vanilla flavor with added protein. Skim milk or a milk alternative provides calcium and additional protein. This dessert is gentle on the digestive system and can be a source of essential nutrients during recovery. The high protein content can help promote satiety and support muscle health. It's a convenient and delicious way to meet protein goals while satisfying your sweet tooth.

Soft Food Phase:

Sugar-Free Greek Yogurt with Berries

Ingredients:

- Low-fat Greek yogurt (unsweetened)

- Fresh berries (e.g., strawberries, blueberries, raspberries)

- Stevia or another sugar substitute (optional)

Step-by-Step Instructions:

1. Start by taking a serving bowl or glass.

2. Measure the desired amount of low-fat Greek yogurt and spoon it into the serving container. The quantity can vary based on your preference, but a typical serving is about 1/2 to 3/4 cup.

3. Wash the fresh berries under cold running water and drain them thoroughly. You can use a mix of berries or choose your favorites.

4. Carefully place the fresh berries on top of the Greek yogurt in the serving container. You can arrange them neatly or simply sprinkle them over the yogurt.

5. If you desire extra sweetness, you can add Stevia or another sugar substitute to the yogurt and berries. The amount depends on your taste, so start with a small amount and adjust as needed.

6. Gently mix the sugar substitute into the yogurt and berries, ensuring it's evenly distributed.

7. Your Sugar-Free Greek Yogurt with Berries is ready to be served. Enjoy it as a healthy and delicious snack or dessert.

Nutritional Information (per serving):

- Calories: Approximately 150-200 calories per serving, depending on the portion size and the use of sugar substitute.

- Protein: Approximately 10-15 grams of protein per serving, primarily from the Greek yogurt.

• Fat: Minimal fat content, mainly from the Greek yogurt.

• Carbohydrates: Approximately 20-30 grams of carbohydrates, primarily from the berries and Greek yogurt.

Low-Sugar Banana Muffins

Ingredients:

• Ripe bananas

• Whole wheat flour

• Unsweetened applesauce

• Stevia or another sugar substitute (optional)

Step-by-Step Instructions:

1. Preheat your oven to 350°F (175°C) and line a muffin tin with paper liners or coat it with non-stick cooking spray.

2. In a mixing bowl, peel and mash the ripe bananas until you have a smooth, lump-free consistency.

3. Add the whole wheat flour and unsweetened applesauce to the mashed bananas. The exact amounts will depend on your desired number of muffins, but as a guideline, use approximately 2 ripe bananas, 1 cup of whole wheat flour, and 1/2 cup of unsweetened applesauce for a small batch. Adjust the quantities as needed to match the number of muffins you wish to make.

4. If you prefer added sweetness, incorporate Stevia or another sugar substitute into the mixture. The amount will vary depending on your taste preference, so start with a small amount and adjust as needed.

5. Mix the ingredients in the bowl thoroughly until you

have a consistent muffin batter. Avoid overmixing; just combine the ingredients until they are incorporated.

6. Spoon the muffin batter into the prepared muffin tin, filling each cup about 2/3 full.

7. Place the muffin tin in the preheated oven and bake for approximately 20-25 minutes or until a toothpick or cake tester inserted into the center of a muffin comes out clean.

8. Once the muffins are done, remove them from the oven and let them cool in the muffin tin for a few minutes.

9. After they have slightly cooled, transfer the muffins to a wire rack to cool completely.

10. Your Low-Sugar Banana Muffins are ready to be enjoyed as a tasty and nutritious snack or breakfast treat.

Portion Sizes:

• The number of muffins produced depends on the size of the muffin tin and how you portion the batter. This recipe typically yields 8-12 muffins.

Cooking Methods:

• The primary cooking method in this recipe is baking in the oven.

Storage and Reheating:

• Store any leftover Low-Sugar Banana Muffins in an airtight container. They can be stored at room temperature for a day or two, or in the refrigerator for longer freshness. Reheat in the microwave for a few seconds or in the oven for a few minutes to enjoy warm.

Nutritional Information (per serving/muffin):

• Calories: Approximately 100-150 calories per muffin, depending on the specific quantities and the use of sugar substitute.

• Protein: Approximately 2-4 grams of protein per muffin, primarily from the whole wheat flour.

• Fat: Minimal fat content, mainly from the unsweetened applesauce.

• Carbohydrates: Approximately 20-25 grams of carbohydrates, primarily from the bananas and whole wheat flour.

Health Benefits:

• Low-Sugar Banana Muffins are a nutritious and low-sugar option suitable for individuals in the post-bariatric surgery phases.

• Ripe bananas provide natural sweetness, fiber, and essential nutrients.

• Whole wheat flour offers whole grains, fiber, and a source of complex carbohydrates.

• Unsweetened applesauce replaces added sugars and contributes to moisture and texture.

• The optional sugar substitute allows for customization without using refined sugars.

• These muffins are gentle on the digestive system, easy to digest, and support recovery and overall health during the post-surgery journey. They are a convenient and satisfying way to enjoy the flavors of banana muffins without excessive added sugars.

Transition to Regular Diet:

Grilled Lemon Chicken

Ingredients:

• Grilled chicken breast

• Lemon juice and zest

• Fresh herbs (e.g., thyme or rosemary)

Step-by-Step Instructions:

1. Preheat your grill to medium-high heat.

2. While the grill is heating up, prepare the lemon marinade. In a mixing bowl, combine fresh lemon juice, lemon zest, and your choice of fresh herbs (e.g., thyme or rosemary). The exact amounts can vary, but a typical marinade for 2 chicken breasts may include the juice and zest of 1 lemon and a few tablespoons of chopped herbs. Adjust the quantities based on your taste.

3. Place the grilled chicken breasts in a shallow dish or a resealable plastic bag.

4. Pour the lemon and herb marinade over the chicken breasts, making sure they are evenly coated. If you're using a plastic bag, seal it and massage the marinade into the chicken to distribute the flavors.

5. Let the chicken marinate for at least 15-30 minutes. For a more intense flavor, you can marinate for up to a few hours in the refrigerator.

6. Once the chicken has marinated, remove it from the dish or bag and allow any excess marinade to drip off.

7. Place the marinated chicken breasts on the preheated grill. Grill each side for approximately 6-8 minutes or until

the internal temperature reaches 165°F (74°C) and the chicken is cooked through.

8. Remove the grilled lemon chicken from the grill and let it rest for a few minutes to allow the juices to redistribute.

9. Slice the grilled lemon chicken and serve it hot, garnished with fresh herbs and lemon wedges if desired.

Portion Sizes:

• The number of servings depends on the number of chicken breasts used. This recipe typically provides 2-4 servings.

Cooking Methods:

• The primary cooking method in this recipe is grilling, which imparts a delightful smoky flavor to the chicken.

Storage and Reheating:

• Store any leftover Grilled Lemon Chicken in an airtight container in the refrigerator. To reheat, gently warm the chicken in the microwave or on the stovetop. Avoid overcooking to maintain the chicken's tenderness.

Nutritional Information (per serving):

• Calories: Approximately 150-200 calories per serving, depending on the portion size and any added fats (e.g., olive oil) in the marinade.

• Protein: Approximately 25-30 grams of protein per serving, primarily from the grilled chicken breast.

• Fat: Minimal fat content, mainly from the marinade.

• Carbohydrates: Minimal carbohydrate content, primarily from the lemon juice and herbs.

Health Benefits:

• Grilled Lemon Chicken is a high-protein, low-fat, and low-carb option suitable for individuals in the post-bariatric surgery phases.

• Grilled chicken breast offers a lean source of protein, which is essential for muscle health and satiety.

• Lemon juice and zest provide a burst of citrusy flavor and vitamin C.

• Fresh herbs not only add flavor but also offer potential health benefits from their natural compounds.

• This dish is easy to digest, promotes satiety, and supports recovery and overall health during the post-surgery journey. It's a flavorful and healthy protein option that can be customized with your choice of herbs and spices.

Mixed Berry Salad with Balsamic Glaze

Ingredients:

• Mixed berries (e.g., strawberries, blueberries, raspberries)

• Balsamic vinegar reduction (sugar-free or low-sugar)

Step-by-Step Instructions:

1. Start by washing and preparing the mixed berries. If using strawberries, remove the stems and slice them. Otherwise, leave the berries whole.

2. In a serving bowl, arrange the mixed berries. You can use a variety of berries to create a colorful and flavorful salad.

3. Drizzle the balsamic vinegar reduction over the mixed berries. The amount you use can vary depending on your taste, but typically 2-3 tablespoons are sufficient for a serving.

4. Gently toss the berries to ensure they are evenly coated with the balsamic glaze. Be careful not to overmix, as berries can be delicate.

5. Your Mixed Berry Salad with Balsamic Glaze is now ready to be served.

Portion Sizes:

• The number of servings depends on the quantity of mixed berries used. This recipe typically provides 2-4 servings.

Cooking Methods:

• This recipe does not involve cooking. It's a no-cook, simple salad.

Storage and Reheating:

• Store any leftover Mixed Berry Salad in the refrigerator. Due to the delicate nature of berries, it's best to consume this salad within a day or two for the best quality. Avoid reheating, as it's intended to be served chilled.

Nutritional Information (per serving):

• Calories: Approximately 50-80 calories per serving, depending on the portion size and the use of balsamic vinegar reduction.

• Protein: Minimal protein content, primarily from the berries.

• Fat: Minimal fat content, primarily from the balsamic vinegar reduction.

• Carbohydrates: Approximately 12-15 grams of carbohydrates per serving, primarily from the mixed berries and balsamic glaze.

Health Benefits:

• Mixed Berry Salad with Balsamic Glaze is a low-calorie, low-fat, and vitamin-rich option suitable for individuals in the post-bariatric surgery phases.

• Mixed berries provide essential vitamins, antioxidants, and dietary fiber.

• Balsamic vinegar reduction adds a sweet and tangy flavor with minimal added sugars.

• This salad is gentle on the digestive system, easy to digest, and supports recovery and overall health during the post-surgery journey. It's a refreshing and nutritious choice that satisfies sweet cravings without excessive sugars. The berries' fiber content can also promote satiety.

CHAPTER 6:

Fiber-Rich Recipes

Clear Liquid Phase:

Clear Broth with Blended Vegetable

Ingredients:

• Low-sodium chicken or vegetable broth

• Steamed and blended zucchini or carrots

Step-by-Step Instructions:

1. Begin by heating the low-sodium chicken or vegetable broth in a saucepan over low to medium heat. The quantity of broth you use depends on the number of servings you want to prepare, but a typical serving is around 1 cup of broth.

2. While the broth is heating, prepare the steamed and blended zucchini or carrots. You can choose either vegetable based on your preference. To do this, steam the zucchini or carrots until they are tender. This can be done by using a steamer, a microwave, or by gently simmering them in water until they are soft.

3. Once the zucchini or carrots are tender, place them in a blender or food processor. Blend until you achieve a smooth puree.

4. Add the vegetable puree to the heated broth. Stir well to combine the two components.

5. Heat the broth and vegetable mixture until it's hot but not boiling.

6. Your Clear Broth with Blended Vegetable is ready to be served. Pour it into a bowl or a cup and enjoy it hot.

Portion Sizes:

• The number of servings depends on the quantity of broth and blended vegetable used. This recipe typically provides 1-2 servings.

Cooking Methods:

• The primary cooking method in this recipe is heating the broth and blending the vegetables.

Storage and Reheating:

• Store any leftover Clear Broth with Blended Vegetable in an airtight container in the refrigerator. Reheat it gently on the stovetop or in the microwave. Avoid boiling to maintain the desired consistency.

Nutritional Information (per serving):

• Calories: Approximately 40-60 calories per serving, depending on the portion size and the type of vegetable used.

• Protein: Approximately 1-2 grams of protein per serving, primarily from the vegetable puree.

• Fat: Minimal fat content, mainly from the vegetable puree.

• Carbohydrates: Approximately 10-15 grams of carbohydrates per serving, primarily from the vegetable puree and broth.

Health Benefits:

• Clear Broth with Blended Vegetable is a low-calorie, low-fat, and easy-to-digest option suitable for individuals in the post-bariatric surgery phases.

• Low-sodium chicken or vegetable broth provides hydration and a gentle base for the soup.

• Steamed and blended zucchini or carrots add vitamins, minerals, and fiber while being easy on the digestive system.

• This soup can provide comfort and nourishment during the early phases of post-surgery recovery, supporting hydration and essential nutrients without overwhelming the digestive tract. It's an ideal choice when more solid foods are not yet recommended.

Mixed Berry Smoothie

Ingredients:

• Frozen mixed berries

• Unflavored protein powder

• Unsweetened almond milk

• A pinch of psyllium husk (for extra fiber)

Step-by-Step Instructions:

1. In a blender, combine a portion of frozen mixed berries. The quantity of berries you use can vary based on your preference, but typically 1 cup of frozen berries makes a single serving.

2. Add one scoop of unflavored protein powder to the blender. You can adjust the quantity based on your protein

needs or preferences.

3. Pour unsweetened almond milk into the blender. The amount can be adjusted to achieve your desired smoothie consistency, but starting with approximately 1 cup is common.

4. Optionally, add a pinch of psyllium husk to the blender. Psyllium husk provides extra dietary fiber, which can aid in digestion and promote a feeling of fullness.

5. Blend all the ingredients until you have a smooth and creamy consistency. If the smoothie is too thick, you can add more almond milk to reach your desired thickness.

6. Pour the mixed berry smoothie into a glass or a portable container, and it's ready to enjoy.

Portion Sizes:

• The number of servings depends on the quantity of ingredients used. This recipe typically provides 1-2 servings.

Cooking Methods:

• This recipe does not involve cooking. It's a simple, no-cook smoothie.

Storage and Reheating:

• You can store any leftover mixed berry smoothie in the refrigerator for a few hours. However, it's best when consumed immediately after preparation.

Nutritional Information (per serving):

• Calories: Approximately 200-250 calories per serving, depending on the portion size and specific ingredients used.

• Protein: Approximately 15-20 grams of protein per

serving, primarily from the protein powder.

• Fat: Minimal fat content, primarily from the almond milk.

• Carbohydrates: Approximately 20-25 grams of carbohydrates per serving, primarily from the mixed berries.

Health Benefits:

• Mixed Berry Smoothie is a convenient and nutritious option suitable for individuals in the post-bariatric surgery phases.

• Frozen mixed berries provide essential vitamins, antioxidants, and natural sweetness.

• Unflavored protein powder ensures that your protein needs are met without added sugars or flavors.

• Unsweetened almond milk offers a creamy base with minimal added sugars.

• Psyllium husk enhances the smoothie's fiber content, promoting satiety and healthy digestion.

• This smoothie is easy to digest, supports recovery and overall health during the post-surgery journey, and serves as a satisfying and refreshing source of essential nutrients. It's an ideal way to increase protein intake while enjoying the flavors of mixed berries.

Full Liquid Phase:

Spinach and Strawberry Protein Smoothie

Ingredients:

• Fresh spinach

• Frozen strawberries

• Unflavored protein powder

• Unsweetened almond milk

Step-by-Step Instructions:

1. Start by washing and preparing the fresh spinach. You can use a handful of fresh spinach leaves, roughly chopped.

2. In a blender, combine the fresh spinach and a portion of frozen strawberries. The exact quantity of strawberries may vary, but typically 1 cup of frozen strawberries makes a single serving.

3. Add one scoop of unflavored protein powder to the blender. Adjust the quantity based on your protein needs or preferences.

4. Pour unsweetened almond milk into the blender. The amount can be adjusted to achieve your desired smoothie consistency, but starting with approximately 1 cup is common.

5. Blend all the ingredients until you have a smooth and creamy consistency. If the smoothie is too thick, you can add more almond milk to reach your desired thickness.

6. Pour the Spinach and Strawberry Protein Smoothie into a glass or a portable container, and it's ready to enjoy.

Portion Sizes:

• The number of servings depends on the quantity of ingredients used. This recipe typically provides 1-2 servings.

Cooking Methods:

• This recipe does not involve cooking. It's a simple, no-cook smoothie.

Storage and Reheating:

• You can store any leftover Spinach and Strawberry Protein Smoothie in the refrigerator for a few hours. However, it's best when consumed immediately after preparation.

Nutritional Information (per serving):

• Calories: Approximately 150-200 calories per serving, depending on the portion size and specific ingredients used.

• Protein: Approximately 15-20 grams of protein per serving, primarily from the protein powder.

• Fat: Minimal fat content, primarily from the almond milk.

• Carbohydrates: Approximately 15-20 grams of carbohydrates per serving, primarily from the strawberries and spinach.

Health Benefits:

• Spinach and Strawberry Protein Smoothie is a nutritious and refreshing option suitable for individuals in the post-bariatric surgery phases.

• Fresh spinach provides vitamins, minerals, and antioxidants, along with dietary fiber.

• Frozen strawberries offer natural sweetness and additional vitamins.

• Unflavored protein powder ensures that your protein needs are met without added sugars or flavors.

• Unsweetened almond milk provides a creamy base with minimal added sugars.

• This smoothie is easy to digest, supports recovery and overall health during the post-surgery journey, and serves as a satisfying source of essential nutrients. It's an ideal way to increase protein intake while enjoying the flavors of spinach and strawberries.

Creamy Butternut Squash Soup

Ingredients:

• Butternut squash, cooked and blended

• Low-sodium vegetable broth

• A pinch of ground flaxseed (for added fiber)

Step-by-Step Instructions:

1. Begin by preparing the butternut squash. You can cook it by roasting, steaming, or microwaving. Once cooked, allow it to cool slightly before proceeding.

2. Cut the cooked butternut squash into chunks and place them in a blender or food processor.

3. Add low-sodium vegetable broth to the blender with the butternut squash. The amount of broth can be adjusted for your desired soup consistency, but starting with approximately 1-2 cups is typical.

4. Optionally, add a pinch of ground flaxseed to the blender. Ground flaxseed is a source of added dietary fiber and can support digestive health.

5. Blend all the ingredients until you achieve a smooth and creamy soup. You can adjust the amount of broth to reach your preferred thickness.

6. Transfer the Creamy Butternut Squash Soup to a pot and heat it over low to medium heat until it's hot but not boiling.

7. Serve the soup in a bowl or a cup, and it's ready to be enjoyed.

Portion Sizes:

• The number of servings depends on the quantity of ingredients used. This recipe typically provides 2-4 servings.

Cooking Methods:

• This recipe involves cooking the butternut squash, but it does not require extensive cooking. It's a blend-and-heat process.

Storage and Reheating:

• Store any leftover Creamy Butternut Squash Soup in the refrigerator. Reheat it gently on the stovetop or in the microwave. Avoid boiling to maintain the desired consistency.

Nutritional Information (per serving):

• Calories: Approximately 80-100 calories per serving, depending on the portion size and specific ingredients used.

• Protein: Minimal protein content, primarily from the vegetable broth.

• Fat: Minimal fat content, primarily from the butternut squash.

• Carbohydrates: Approximately 20-25 grams of carbohydrates per serving, primarily from the butternut squash.

Health Benefits:

• Creamy Butternut Squash Soup is a low-calorie and nutrient-rich choice suitable for individuals in the post-bariatric surgery phases.

• Butternut squash provides essential vitamins, minerals,

and dietary fiber, making it a nutritious addition to your diet.

• Low-sodium vegetable broth offers a flavorful base for the soup.

• Ground flaxseed adds extra dietary fiber, supporting digestive health and promoting satiety.

• This soup is gentle on the digestive system, easy to digest, and supports recovery and overall health during the post-surgery journey. It's a warming and nourishing option that is both comforting and nutritious.

Pureed Food Phase:

Mashed Sweet Potatoes and Carrots

Ingredients:

• Cooked sweet potatoes and carrots (blended)

• A pinch of chia seeds (for added fiber)

• A drizzle of olive oil (in moderation)

Step-by-Step Instructions:

1. Start by cooking the sweet potatoes and carrots. You can cook them by boiling, roasting, or steaming until they are tender. Once cooked, allow them to cool slightly before proceeding.

2. Cut the cooked sweet potatoes and carrots into chunks and place them in a blender or food processor.

3. Blend the sweet potatoes and carrots until you achieve a smooth and creamy consistency. You can adjust the texture by adding a small amount of water or vegetable broth if needed.

4. Add a pinch of chia seeds to the blended mixture. Chia

seeds are a great source of dietary fiber and can enhance the nutritional content.

5. Optionally, drizzle a small amount of olive oil over the mashed sweet potatoes and carrots. Use it in moderation for added flavor and healthy fats.

6. Mix the chia seeds and olive oil into the mashed sweet potatoes and carrots until well combined.

7. Serve the Mashed Sweet Potatoes and Carrots as a side dish or enjoy them as a standalone meal.

Portion Sizes:

• The number of servings depends on the quantity of ingredients used. This recipe typically provides 2-4 servings.

Cooking Methods:

• This recipe involves cooking the sweet potatoes and carrots and then blending them. It's a blend-and-enhance process.

Storage and Reheating:

• Store any leftover Mashed Sweet Potatoes and Carrots in an airtight container in the refrigerator. Reheat them gently in the microwave or on the stovetop. Add a small amount of water or broth if they have thickened during storage.

Nutritional Information (per serving):

• Calories: Approximately 80-120 calories per serving, depending on the portion size and specific ingredients used.

• Protein: Minimal protein content, primarily from the chia seeds.

• Fat: Approximately 3-5 grams of fat per serving, mainly from the olive oil.

• Carbohydrates: Approximately 15-20 grams of carbohydrates per serving, primarily from the sweet potatoes and carrots.

Health Benefits:

• Mashed Sweet Potatoes and Carrots are a flavorful and nutritious choice suitable for individuals in the post-bariatric surgery phases.

• Sweet potatoes and carrots provide essential vitamins, minerals, and dietary fiber, making this dish both nutritious and satisfying.

• Chia seeds add extra dietary fiber, supporting digestive health and promoting a feeling of fullness.

• Olive oil, when used in moderation, contributes healthy monounsaturated fats and a pleasant flavor.

• This dish is easy to digest, supports recovery and overall health during the post-surgery journey, and offers a delicious way to incorporate essential nutrients into your diet. It's a comforting and wholesome option for bariatric patients.

Black Bean Puree

Ingredients:

• Canned black beans, drained and blended

• A pinch of ground cumin

• Fresh cilantro (optional)

Step-by-Step Instructions:

1. Start by draining and rinsing the canned black beans. This helps reduce the sodium content.

2. Place the drained black beans in a blender or food processor.

3. Add a pinch of ground cumin to the beans. Cumin provides a warm and earthy flavor that pairs well with black beans.

4. Optionally, you can incorporate fresh cilantro for added flavor. Fresh cilantro can enhance the taste and aroma of the puree.

5. Blend the ingredients until you achieve a smooth and creamy consistency. You may need to add a small amount of water to reach your desired texture.

6. Once blended, taste the puree and adjust the seasoning if necessary. You can add more cumin or cilantro according to your preference.

7. Serve the Black Bean Puree as a side dish or use it as a topping for lean proteins or vegetables.

Portion Sizes:

• The number of servings depends on the quantity of ingredients used. This recipe typically provides 2-4 servings.

Cooking Methods:

• This recipe is a no-cook option, making it easy to prepare.

Storage and Reheating:

• Store any leftover Black Bean Puree in an airtight container in the refrigerator. Reheat it gently in the microwave or on the stovetop. Add a small amount of water if it has thickened during storage.

Nutritional Information (per serving):

• Calories: Approximately 60-80 calories per serving, depending on the portion size and specific ingredients used.

• Protein: Approximately 3-5 grams of protein per serving, primarily from the black beans.

• Fat: Minimal fat content.

• Carbohydrates: Approximately 12-15 grams of carbohydrates per serving, primarily from the black beans.

Health Benefits:

• Black Bean Puree is a protein-rich and nutritious choice suitable for individuals in the post-bariatric surgery phases.

• Black beans are an excellent source of plant-based protein, fiber, vitamins, and minerals.

• Ground cumin adds flavor and has potential health benefits, including digestion support and antioxidant properties.

• Fresh cilantro enhances the taste and provides a burst of freshness.

• This puree is easy to digest, supports recovery and overall health during the post-surgery journey, and offers a flavorful and wholesome option for bariatric patients.

Soft Food Phase:

Quinoa and Vegetable Stir-Fry

Ingredients:

• Cooked quinoa

• Mixed stir-fry vegetables (e.g., bell peppers, broccoli)

• Low-sodium soy sauce (in moderation)

Step-by-Step Instructions:

1. Begin by cooking quinoa according to the package instructions. Quinoa typically requires 15-20 minutes to cook, but check the package for specific directions.

2. While the quinoa is cooking, prepare your stir-fry vegetables. Wash and cut them into bite-sized pieces. Common choices include bell peppers, broccoli, carrots, and snap peas, but feel free to customize your selection.

3. In a non-stick skillet or wok, heat a small amount of water or cooking spray over medium-high heat.

4. Add the prepared vegetables to the skillet. Stir-fry them for 3-5 minutes or until they are tender and slightly crisp.

5. Once the quinoa is cooked and the vegetables are tender, combine the cooked quinoa and stir-fried vegetables in the skillet. Mix them well to ensure an even distribution.

6. Drizzle low-sodium soy sauce over the quinoa and vegetables. Use soy sauce in moderation to control the sodium content.

7. Continue to stir-fry for an additional 2-3 minutes, allowing the flavors to meld and the soy sauce to coat the ingredients evenly.

8. Taste the stir-fry and adjust the seasoning if necessary.

You can add more soy sauce if desired.

9. Serve the Quinoa and Vegetable Stir-Fry as a balanced and satisfying meal.

Portion Sizes:

• The number of servings depends on the quantity of ingredients used. This recipe typically provides 2-4 servings.

Cooking Methods:

• This recipe involves cooking quinoa and stir-frying vegetables. It's a straightforward process.

Storage and Reheating:

• Store any leftover Quinoa and Vegetable Stir-Fry in an airtight container in the refrigerator. Reheat it gently in the microwave or on the stovetop. Add a small amount of water if it has dried out during storage.

Nutritional Information (per serving):

• Calories: Approximately 150-200 calories per serving, depending on the portion size and specific ingredients used.

• Protein: Approximately 5-8 grams of protein per serving, primarily from quinoa and vegetables.

• Fat: Minimal fat content.

• Carbohydrates: Approximately 25-30 grams of carbohydrates per serving, primarily from quinoa and vegetables.

Health Benefits:

• Quinoa and Vegetable Stir-Fry is a balanced and nutritious choice suitable for individuals in the post-bariatric surgery phases.

• Quinoa is a high-quality source of plant-based protein, and it's also rich in fiber, vitamins, and minerals.

• Mixed vegetables provide essential nutrients and dietary fiber, promoting overall health.

• Low-sodium soy sauce adds flavor without excessive salt, making it a heart-healthy option.

• This dish is easy to digest, supports recovery and weight management during the post-surgery journey, and offers a tasty and wholesome option for bariatric patients.

Fruit and Yogurt Parfait

Ingredients:

• Low-fat Greek yogurt (unsweetened)

• Fresh berries

• Chopped nuts (in moderation) for added crunch and fiber

Step-by-Step Instructions:

1. Begin by selecting a glass or a small bowl in which you'll assemble your parfait.

2. Start by adding a layer of low-fat Greek yogurt to the bottom of the glass or bowl. The amount can vary based on your preference, but a 1/2 cup of yogurt is a common serving size.

3. Wash and prepare your choice of fresh berries. Common options include strawberries, blueberries, raspberries, and blackberries. You can use one type of berry or a mixture of your favorites.

4. Add a layer of fresh berries on top of the yogurt. This

provides natural sweetness and vibrant colors to your parfait.

5. Optionally, sprinkle a small amount of chopped nuts over the berries. Nuts add a delightful crunch and provide healthy fats and fiber. Use them in moderation to control portion size.

6. Repeat the layers by adding more yogurt, berries, and nuts until you've used up your ingredients or reached your desired portion.

7. Finish your parfait with a final drizzle of yogurt and a few fresh berries on top for an attractive presentation.

8. Your Fruit and Yogurt Parfait is ready to enjoy.

Portion Sizes:

• The number of servings depends on the quantity of ingredients used. This recipe typically provides 1-2 servings.

Cooking Methods:

• This recipe involves no cooking; it's an assembly process.

Storage and Reheating:

• Parfaits are best enjoyed fresh. However, if you need to store any leftovers, cover the glass or bowl with plastic wrap and refrigerate. Consume within a day for optimal freshness.

Nutritional Information (per serving):

• Calories: Approximately 150-200 calories per serving, depending on the portion size and specific ingredients used.

• Protein: Approximately 10-15 grams of protein per serving, primarily from Greek yogurt and nuts.

• Fat: Approximately 5-8 grams of fat per serving, mainly from nuts and yogurt.

• Carbohydrates: Approximately 20-30 grams of carbohydrates per serving, primarily from the berries and yogurt.

Health Benefits:

• Fruit and Yogurt Parfait is a nutrient-dense and protein-rich choice suitable for individuals in the post-bariatric surgery phases.

• Low-fat Greek yogurt provides a good source of protein, calcium, and probiotics for gut health.

• Fresh berries offer vitamins, antioxidants, and dietary fiber, supporting overall well-being.

• Chopped nuts, when used in moderation, supply healthy fats, protein, and fiber, adding a delightful crunch.

• This parfait is easy to digest, aids recovery, and makes a satisfying and flavorful option for bariatric patients. It's a tasty way to incorporate essential nutrients into your diet.

Transition to Regular Diet:

Chicken and Brown Rice Soup

Ingredients:

• Cooked chicken breast, shredded

• Cooked brown rice

• Mixed vegetables (e.g., carrots, peas)

• Low-sodium chicken broth

Step-by-Step Instructions:

1. Start by preparing the ingredients. Ensure that the

chicken breast is cooked and shredded, the brown rice is cooked, and the mixed vegetables are ready.

2. In a large soup pot, pour the low-sodium chicken broth. The amount of broth depends on how much soup you intend to make, but a standard serving often includes 1-2 cups of broth.

3. Heat the chicken broth over medium heat until it starts to simmer.

4. Add the shredded cooked chicken breast and mixed vegetables to the simmering broth. The vegetables can be a combination of carrots and peas, but you can adjust the selection to your preference.

5. Allow the soup to cook for 5-10 minutes, or until the vegetables become tender. Cooking time may vary based on the size of the vegetable pieces.

6. Once the vegetables are tender, add the cooked brown rice to the soup. Stir well to incorporate all the ingredients.

7. Simmer the soup for an additional 5-10 minutes, allowing the flavors to meld together.

8. Taste the soup and adjust the seasoning if necessary. You can add a pinch of salt or pepper, but it's best to use seasonings in moderation to control sodium content.

9. Your Chicken and Brown Rice Soup is now ready to serve.

Portion Sizes:

• The number of servings depends on the quantity of ingredients used. This recipe typically provides 2-4 servings.

Cooking Methods:

• This recipe involves stovetop cooking and is a simple and

convenient process.

Storage and Reheating:

• Store any leftover Chicken and Brown Rice Soup in an airtight container in the refrigerator. Reheat it gently in the microwave or on the stovetop. Add a small amount of water if it has thickened during storage.

Nutritional Information (per serving):

• Calories: Approximately 150-200 calories per serving, depending on the portion size and specific ingredients used.

• Protein: Approximately 15-20 grams of protein per serving, primarily from chicken and brown rice.

• Fat: Minimal fat content.

• Carbohydrates: Approximately 20-30 grams of carbohydrates per serving, mainly from brown rice and vegetables.

Health Benefits:

• Chicken and Brown Rice Soup is a balanced and nutritious choice suitable for individuals in the post-bariatric surgery phases.

• Cooked chicken breast provides lean protein, while brown rice offers fiber and complex carbohydrates.

• Mixed vegetables contribute essential nutrients, vitamins, and dietary fiber.

• Low-sodium chicken broth enhances flavor while helping control salt intake.

• This soup is easy to digest, supports recovery, and provides a wholesome and satisfying option for bariatric patients. It's a warm and comforting meal, perfect for post-surgery nourishment.

Grilled Shrimp and Asparagus

Ingredients:

• Grilled shrimp

• Fresh asparagus spears

• Quinoa or brown rice (cooked)

Step-by-Step Instructions:

1. Start by preparing the ingredients. Ensure the shrimp is already grilled, the asparagus is washed and trimmed, and the quinoa or brown rice is cooked and ready.

2. Preheat your grill or grill pan to medium-high heat.

3. While the grill is heating, you can season the shrimp and asparagus as desired. A light drizzle of olive oil, a pinch of salt and pepper, and a sprinkle of your favorite herbs or seasonings work well.

4. Place the seasoned shrimp and asparagus on the grill. Shrimp usually cook quickly, so be attentive. Grill for about 2–3 minutes per side until they turn pink and opaque.

5. The asparagus may take a bit longer, typically 5-7 minutes, depending on their thickness. Grill them until they become tender with some charred marks.

6. As the shrimp and asparagus cook, reheat the cooked

quinoa or brown rice either on the stovetop or in the microwave. Fluff it with a fork.

7. Once the shrimp, asparagus, and grain are ready, assemble your meal. Place a serving of quinoa or brown rice on your plate, top it with grilled shrimp, and arrange the grilled asparagus alongside.

8. Your grilled shrimp and asparagus dish is now ready to enjoy.

Portion Sizes:

• The number of servings depends on the quantity of ingredients used. This recipe typically provides 2-4 servings.

Cooking Methods:

• Grilling is the primary cooking method for this dish, but you'll also need to reheat the cooked quinoa or brown rice.

Storage and Reheating:

• Any leftovers can be stored in airtight containers in the refrigerator. Reheat them gently in the microwave or on the stovetop. Add a splash of water if the grains have dried out during storage.

Nutritional information (per serving):

• Calories: approximately 200–250 calories per serving, depending on the portion size and specific ingredients used.

• Protein: Approximately 20–25 grams of protein per serving, primarily from shrimp.

• Fat: minimal fat content, especially if you use a light drizzle of olive oil.

• Carbohydrates: Approximately 20–30 grams of

carbohydrates per serving, mainly from quinoa, brown rice, and asparagus.

Health Benefits:

• Grilled shrimp and asparagus is a protein-rich and balanced option suitable for individuals in the post-bariatric surgery phases.

• Shrimp offers a lean source of protein, asparagus contributes vitamins and fiber, and quinoa or brown rice provides complex carbohydrates and additional fiber.

• This dish is easy to digest, supports recovery, and is a flavorful and wholesome choice for bariatric patients. It's an excellent way to include essential nutrients in your post-surgery diet.

CONCLUSION

In closing, this Gastric Sleeve Bariatric Cookbook has been crafted with the utmost care to guide you on your post-surgery journey towards better health and well-being. Throughout these pages, you've discovered a variety of delicious and nourishing recipes, along with valuable insights into the phases of recovery following gastric sleeve surgery.

The key takeaways from this cookbook are centered on nourishment, balance, and mindfulness. You've learned how to embrace a diet that supports your healing process while also promoting weight loss and long-term health. From clear liquids to soft foods and eventually to regular solid foods, the transition has been made more accessible, and fiber, protein, and low-sugar options have been thoughtfully integrated into your meal plans.

But beyond the recipes and dietary guidelines, remember that your post-surgery journey is a unique and transformative one. It's a path towards better health, newfound confidence, and a brighter future. There will be moments of challenge, but within every challenge lies an opportunity for growth and perseverance.

So, as you continue on your post-surgery path, I encourage you to stay committed to the healthy choices you've discovered in these pages. Seek support from your healthcare team, dietitian, and loved ones. Embrace mindful eating and find joy in savoring each meal. You are not alone in this journey, and success is within reach.

Every step you take, every meal you savor, and every healthy choice you make brings you closer to a vibrant and fulfilling life. Your journey is a testament to your strength, resilience, and determination, and the reward is a healthier, happier you.

May this cookbook serve as a guiding light on your path, and may you find comfort, nourishment, and a world of flavors to explore as you continue your remarkable journey towards a healthier, more vibrant you. Remember, you've got this, and the future is filled with endless possibilities.